THE EASY LOW-COST WAY TO TOTAL BEAUTY

THE EASY LOW-COST WAY TO TOTAL BEAUTY

By
LELORD KORDEL

G. P. PUTNAM'S SONS
NEW YORK, N.Y.

 Published simultaneously in Canada
by Longman Canada Limited, Toronto.

SBN: 399-11914-0

Library of Congress Cataloging in Publication Data

Kordel, Lelord.
The easy low-cost way to total beauty.

1. Beauty, Personal. I. Title.
RA778.K7255 1979 646.7 78-15816

PRINTED IN THE UNITED STATES OF AMERICA

to Verdice—
the beautiful lady in my life

CONTENTS

THE EASY LOW-COST WAY TO TOTAL BEAUTY

Chapter I

THE MULTI-BILLION DOLLAR BEAUTY RIPOFF

"Want the very best cosmetic you can get?

"Just place a drop of Chanel No. 5 in a can of bear grease and you'll have a cosmetic cream as good as any on the market today.

"Or stir your favorite scent into petroleum jelly or beeswax. Add a little water (or alcohol) to thin it, and you'll have the same results as that $20-per-ounce, commercially manufactured 'skin rejuvenator' decorating the cosmetic shelf. It smells good and retains natural body moisture."

This advice, strange as it seems, did not come from an avid do-it-yourself-er who resides in the deepest jungles of Peru. Nor from a nomad wandering around the Gobi Desert. Nor did it come from an isolated seal hunter in Alaska.

It was an off-the-record statement made to me during an interview several years ago with a prominent cosmetic scientist. It is understandable why he wishes to remain anonymous.

But his statement did inspire the researcher in me to begin a lifelong study into not only what ladies put on the inside of them ... but also, what they put on the *outside* of them. One most definitely affects the other.

"Of course, if one misses the 'eye-appeal'—the aesthetics—of cosmetic packaging," the cosmetic scientist continued, "just place this homemade mixture into your most elegant decanter and—*voilà*—you have a snob-appeal cosmetic product equal to any available, whether imported or domestic."

Recently, while shopping in a well-known New York department store, I found myself meandering through the toiletries and cosmetics section. This experience was mind-boggling.

Before me stretched aisle upon aisle of counters, each displaying a mass of eye makeups, skin treatments, hair conditioners, and an endless array of other products claiming the power to make women more beautiful. Though their formulas were many and varied, they all shared one common denominator: *high cost.*

There was one product referred to as a "hydracel toner" and another described as "tissular cream." Depending on the money a woman was willing to spend, she could invest in a "rich whipped cleanser" or in an "eye cream plus" or perhaps in a "Swiss performing extract."

I discovered, too, that price is proportional to the amount of French in a product's description. Hence, *"formule spéciale"* competed with *"tonique douceur."* Instead of ordinary moisturizers one counter displayed a whoppingly expensive *"crème de nuit adoucissement"* while another offered a skin compound described as *"traitement exfoliant pour le corps."*

No wonder they're so costly, with all the extra expense that goes into typesetting!

But it didn't stop there. At many of the displays stood charming young ladies—some young enough to be my granddaughters—all passing themselves off as "experts" or "consultants." Among those I questioned, their credentials consisted of little more than a few weeks' basic training in a vague school or company course.

Whatever, there these lovely young wizardesses stood, dispensing the benefits of their questionable sagacity or applying the proper product to fit the individual consumer's needs. Strangely, each seemed to have her own favorite cosmetics—all of which, by some fortuitous coincidence, came from the same manufacturer or distributor.

It's strange how women allow themselves to be hypnotized into buying more and more of these astronomically priced beauty products when they can make an even better product at home for a fraction of the cost.

"So what?" many of you ask. "These are modern times. If we can afford little luxuries to help keep us beautiful, why shouldn't we indulge ourselves?"

Why indeed? Because with every high-priced cosmetic purchase you are also buying dyes, fixatives, preservatives, and a host of other properties—none of which are beautifying and many of which could be downright dangerous.

Moreover, about 50 percent of the price goes for advertising and packaging. Plus, frequently, a substantial proportion pays off the fashion designer or celebrity whose name is used to promote the product.

The addition of anything exotic or scientific sounding, whether its benefits have been proved or not, seems to be all it takes to turn a one-dollar cream into one that will sell for twenty. Hard-sell advertising can actually convince many women that twenty dollars' worth of cream must be twenty times as potent as the cheaper one. A conviction the cosmetic companies foster and count on!

This conviction is carefully nurtured in all areas of cosmetics. Perhaps the most blatant example is lipsticks. I will always remember how my friend George Corbin, a chemist by profession, blew his top when his wife bought a very expensive lipstick. "How many times do I have to remind you?" he shouted. "Lipstick is lipstick! There is only one way to make it. You just paid for a fancy case and perfume. If you must wear the stuff, buy it in the variety store."

When he calmed down, George explained that "cheaper" lipsticks are basically the same as expensive brands. The bigger cosmetic companies put extra money into packaging, even to the extent of calling in a jewelry designer to create a new lipstick container. Then the cost of the design is added to the price. Nothing is added to the basic formula, which has probably been the same since they went into business. And regardless of cost, lipstick, like all cosmetics, must conform to governmental purity standards.

In fact, most cosmetic items contain the same emollient bases—emollients that can be purchased in any drugstore at very reasonable prices. Some are thicker, some thinner, some colored darker, some lighter. Differently packaged, scented, and priced but basically the same, except of course for the chemical additives and preservatives and doubtful "miracle" ingredients.

Sometimes the containers are more expensive than the product plus miracle ingredient. Often the perfumes used are more expensive than everything combined. But perfume adds nothing to the effectiveness of a cream or lotion; it only adds to the price.

A leading dermatologist, Dr. Bedford Shelmire, Jr., of the Univeristy of Texas Southwestern Medical School, gave this opinion of overpriced cosmetics and the additives they contain:

"Usually the more expensive the beauty product, the more problems it causes. The additives they put in not only increase the cost, but can cause skin irritation. And when a product is advertised as *New and Improved,* it generally means that new chemicals have been added to it and that the consumer will pay more for it."

Perhaps the most flagrant and cynical consumer traps are the overblown promotions for "rare, precious, and costly" ingredients that instantly raise the price of a jar of any cosmetic.

Inspired, no doubt, by the high price of a mink coat, manufacturers turned to mink oil as a miracle skin rejuvenator. Advertising brought the price of an ounce of mink oil hand cream to $12.50. But mink oil has proved to have no value, except to give the product snob appeal and keep prices on the rise.

After animal oils became a drag on the market, cosmeticians turned back the clock and rediscovered—milk! The way one manufacturer told it, milk was a trend-setting discovery. He conveniently forgot that milk baths go back to antiquity and that nutritionists have stressed the benefits of milk for many years.

Another milk-containing cosmetic listed a preservative on the label. Of course, something had to keep the milk fresh. So what they were selling was six ounces of preserved milk for $4. Ridiculous, when thirty-two ounces of fresh milk still sell for under a dollar . . . and if you don't use all of it on your skin, you can drink the rest.

Always on the hunt for miracle ingredients, in the 1960s cosmeticians came up with a rash of "temporary wrinkle smoothers," all of them containing something called "bovine serum albumin" which translates into—protein from cattle blood. Even more unaesthetic were the creams and lotions with placental extracts and embryonic fluids. These rather strange preparations may have been beneficial to human and animal embryos, but proved to be entirely useless in cosmetics.

Inevitably, we come to the obvious question: *how does the cosmetic consumer avoid getting ripped off?* The answer: *become your own comparison shopper.*

You can get the most for your money simply by reading labels—not just for brand names and slick slogans but also for ingredients. Only then will you begin to appreciate this admonition from the former director of a large cosmetics firm:

"There is no difference in basic ingredients between high- and low-priced cosmetics. The same company might be selling a cheap face cream and an expensive one, and they would be exactly the same except for fragrance. All cosmetic firms use the same basic ingredients."

There is also value to be gained by reading the directions on a product's label. Often, with some simple arithmetic, you'll find that it does pay to spend a few pennies more if you use less of a product each time you apply it. Frequency is also significant: a cream applied once a day will last twice as long as a cream applied twice a day.

Finally you should determine a cosmetic's "life span" before making your purchase. This is especially true of eye makeup and skin cream, which can spoil or turn rancid on your shelf. If the label doesn't indicate how long a product may be safely kept, then write to the manufacturer and request such information. And while awaiting his reply, ask yourself what he is trying to hide!

Armed with these helpful hints, are you now ready to do battle with the cosmetics market without fear of being ripped off? Not by a long shot!

The almighty dollar is only one side of the cosmetics picture. In the next chapter, you will discover a far greater crime committed by manufacturers: the rip-off of your health and well-being.

Chapter II

BEAUTY— AT WHAT SACRIFICE?

The scene is your local department store, pharmacy, or supermarket. Arrayed on the shelves are myriad shampoos, hair rinses, skin creams, eye shadows. Some are plainly packaged, with prices that won't harm your budget. Others are fancily encased, have exotic names, and sell at three, five, or ten times the amount.

On this trip, you're resolved not to be conned by fluffery and frills. You will study the labels and determine which is the best buy. How can you go wrong?

You reach for the first bottle, and what do you discover? Among its ingredients are *glyceryl stearate, aluminum chlorohydrate* and *cetyl alcohol.* Now you know what you're paying for, right? Wrong . . . unless you're a graduate chemist.

Maybe another bottle will be easier to decipher. You search the fine print until you're able to make out the jawbreaker, *methyl and propylparahydroxy-benzoates.*

Somehow you're feeling more helpless than when you started.

Try one more ... ah, here's a beauty: *sodium laurel sulfate, hydroxyethylcellulose, polystyrene copolymer!*

For the first time you realize a frightening fact. Not only don't you know if you're getting your money's worth—you may also be dousing your hair, shading your eyes, or coating your skin with potentially dangerous chemicals.

If this sounds alarmist, let's simplify the picture with some terms that are more familiar to you.

Formaldehyde. Chloroform. Sodium hydroxide. Potassium hydroxide. Do they sound like ingredients on the shelves of your neighborhood exterminator? Some of them probably are, but did you know that they may also be found in the cosmetics you use every day on your face, hair, and body?

In pursuit of the dollar, pound, peso, franc, and whatever form of currency is available, the cosmetics industry goes on its merry way using ingredients without concern for their possible long-range effects as irritants, poisons—or both. Any way you look at it, the consumer is taking chances.

That highly touted shampoo which "leaves your hair silky and shining" may cause serious damage if it gets into your eyes. There are warnings on shampoo labels, but people do slip up when washing their hair. What happens then? Irritation? Redness and swelling? Permanent damage to the delicate membranes?

For many women, cosmetics are as much a part of everyday life as eating, breathing, and sleeping. But did you realize that until very recently cosmetics were the only products *not* required to list active ingredients?

With most everything, you are told exactly what you are buying. For years, ingredients and additives in foods have been printed on the labels. Drug elements are not only listed, but possible side effects are noted. In clothing, everything from undershirts to scarves carries a label noting the fibers in the fabric and how to clean them.

But anything called a "cosmetic" was getting into the marketplace after a minimum of testing or no testing at all. Cosmetic companies balked at disclosing ingredients because, they insisted, there are too many to list on small labels. Besides, they pleaded, if they were forced to reveal secret formulas, competitors would be able to duplicate their "miracle" ingredients. Could it be that they were worried that some consumers might decipher what those ingredients actually were?

When I made this point about cosmetics at a friend's home one evening, his wife brought out a bottle of something labeled "All-Purpose Body Lotion" to show me that the ingredients were indeed listed. There they were, all eleven of them and all sounding very scientific. An imposing array of names that few laymen could decipher.

One compound immediately caught my eye: sodium hydroxide, a caustic substance used in textile finishing and bleaching—and an important ingredient in solutions the plumber uses to unstop clogged drains.

A look at *The United States Pharmacopeia* shows this notation under sodium hydroxide: *"Caution—exercise great care in handling, as it rapidly destroys tissues."*

Disturbing, isn't it? What is it doing in a body lotion?

Unless you carry a dictionary or a copy of the pharmacopeia under your arm on shopping trips, you still won't know exactly what you are buying in that pretty bottle. Labeling has convinced the public that if the ingredients are listed, they must be pure and safe.

But are they?

Today's world of cosmetics consists of more than

lipstick and paint. Almost everything you use daily to powder and pamper yourself is included—toothpaste, shampoo, baby oil, shaving cream, deodorants, nail polish. The list even contains items that don't fit into other categories—such as scented toilet tissue, which, incidentally, has been responsible for rashes and inflammations of the rectal and genital area.

As defined by law, cosmetics are: "Articles intended to be rubbed, poured, sprinkled, or sprayed on, introduced into, or otherwise applied to the human body or any part thereof for cleansing, beautifying, promoting attractiveness, or altering the appearance ..."

Under the circumstances, one might expect that cosmetics be required to meet the same standards and safeguards as food and drugs. Unfortunately, government watchdogs can only get into the act if there are reports of damage or injury related to the use of a cosmetic.

Where does that leave you, the consumer? Even though a product may do no harm, can you be certain it is really safe?

Until a few years ago, the whole family was virtually saturated from sunup to sundown with a product called hexachlorophene. In TV commercials, in magazine and newspaper ads, white-coated "scientists" extolled its virtues, while housewives and models, lawyers and athletes confirmed its benefits. Hexachlorophene, a disinfectant and germicide, was included in everything from creams, lotions, mouthwash, and shaving products to hair preparations, makeup and, of course, "intimate" sprays.

In those so-called intimate sprays, hexachlorophene was responsible for many irritations of the nether regions of people who should have known that frequent applications of soap and water would have been far more efficient. But advertising had almost everyone convinced that hexachlorophene was good for them. So good, in fact, that many wondered how they had managed to live without it all these years.

Then reports began to filter through that hexachlorophene was causing serious damage to infants bathed with it. Some suffered convulsions and brain damage. Further tests showed that it was absorbed through the skin and could actually be measured in the blood.

Finally in 1972 the manufacture of products containing hexachlorophene was banned. One less ingredient to worry about.

Ammoniated mercury, also capable of poisoning the body by absorption through the skin, was a basic ingredient of "bleaching" and "skin toner" creams for many years. In late 1972 growing reports of systemic poisonings from use of these creams finally forced their reclassification as drugs—which made the listing of ingredients and hazard warnings a "must."

As an example of how poisonous ammoniated mercury really is, a number of regulatory agencies forced the suspension of all commercial fishing on the Great Lakes when it was learned that industrial wastes containing mercury were being dumped into these lakes. Imagine—after being diluted by billions of gallons of water, the mercury was still sufficiently potent to harm humans who consumed fish caught in these lakes.

To keep his product from becoming a drug, one large manufacturer gave up ammoniated mercury and changed to his own trademarked ingredient, which he listed on the label. That ingredient turned out to be hydroquinone.

Have you ever heard of hydroquinone? According to the *Merck Index*, the cosmetics-trade reference book, hydroquinone is "relatively safe in very low concentrations." The index goes on to say that one of its uses is as a photographic reducer and developer, and that dermatitis can result from skin contact. As to toxic effects, it can cause nausea, convulsions, delirium. A case of the manufacturer showing his concern for the consumer by switching from one poison to another!

When they switch to "miracle" ingredients, the cosmetics purveyors usually go all the way. Several years ago, pseudo-scientific promotions touted the benefits of estrogen in cosmetics. Posing amid test tubes and laboratory equipment, cosmeticians made fantastic claims about "soft, youthful skin" obtained with estrogenic hormone preparations.

Dr. Howard Behrman, director of dermatological research at New York Medical College, has stated categorically that hormone creams do nothing for the skin. In fact, estrogens can be absorbed through the skin to upset the body's hormone balance and in some instances create symptoms similar to those of cancer.

Thousands of chemical compounds are being used in the manufacture of cosmetics. Each year hundreds more are added to the list. Like hexachlorophene, the harmful ones may not be discovered until years later—after they have done an alarming amount of damage.

How does this affect you as a consumer? Once again, you must approach your purchases with patience and a wary eye. You stand a better chance of protecting yourself if you learn to read labels.

A label should state that the product has been tested for safety by the manufacturer before going on sale.

If you tend to have allergies, or just to be on the safe side, aim for the product whose label clearly states: *hypoallergenic.* This simply means that it is less likely to produce an allergic reaction. However, it is not a guarantee.

When in doubt about your allergic response to a product, don't use it until you've tested it. This can be done by applying a small amount to the side of your forearm and leaving it on for twenty-four hours. In the event of any redness, blistering, burning or itching, get rid of the cosmetic—you're allergic to something in it.

Unfortunately, labels don't tell you everything you need to know. In order to do a thorough job of protecting yourself, write to the manufacturer about specific chemical ingredients that concern you.

By all means, you want to avoid the *four major poisons* that pop up in cosmetics: *zinc, lead, copper, mercury.*

Then there are contaminants that may result from incomplete chemical reactions during manufacture—acetones, aldehydes, alkalis—plus caustic volatile oils and coal-tar derivatives. Are they present or aren't they? And in what percentage? Only the manufacturer knows for sure.

The cautious cosmetics consumer is far better able to guard her health and budget than the frivolous, gullible buyer. But for near-perfect protection—without having to read labels or write to manufacturers—there's a much surer approach in the chapters ahead.

Chapter III

NATURE'S WAY TO BEAUTY

Dorothy Parker, author and wit, once wrote: "Imagine that the huge amounts of money American men and women spend annually on hand cream, face lotion, anti-wrinkle emollients, skin 'dew' and thousands of other such preparations were devoted to a propaganda campaign pushing the importance of proper nutrition; the cosmetics industry would collapse, but the general condition of human hides would be vastly improved."

Was the sharp-tongued Ms. Parker referring to the face and bath powders that usually contain pulverized rock or metal? Perhaps she herself suffered allergies that surfaced from the dyes and fixatives added to rouge, lipsticks, and eye shadows. Or was she warning about the chlorides and sulfates in commercial deodorants, the hormones and caustic ingredients in skin preparations—all suspected of producing rashes, irritations, and even cancer.

These are serious risks. Are they worth taking? *Must*

you take them in order to remain beautiful and sexually stimulating?

Women have been concerned with their allure through every age of history, but only in modern times have they been bombarded with such a bewildering assortment of commercial beauty products.

Egyptian ladies were famous for accenting their eyes and reddening their hair. Among *les femmes* of the French court, powder, rouge, and beauty marks were the vogue.

But without access to cosmetics manufacturers, all the sirens of the past as far back as Cleopatra relied on nature's pure and unadulterated products to brew their beauty aids.

Of course Cleopatra herself didn't stand over the hot cooking pots. More likely she relied on a handmaiden to attend to the stirring and simmering, while still another was out gathering the plants, herbs, roots, and leaves that were the ingredients of Cleopatra's cosmetic recipes—recipes that remained in use for several thousand years. Henna, a vegetable dye used by Egyptian ladies to tint their hair a bright auburn, is still in use today.

Another enchantress of long ago, Ninon de Lenclos, proved that age is no barrier to beauty. Historians have stated that her youthful appearance had young men falling in love with her when she was seventy years old! Her secret was also from nature—a secret she probably did not share with the other ladies of the French court. She did all her bathing in a combination of several herbs.

However, in talking about natural cosmetics I need not go so far into history. My grandmother and her mother prized their secret beauty recipes brewed from nature's products. Some of their ingredients were often taken from the kitchen shelves. I remember how proud my grandmother was of her soft skin and creamy complexion—a complexion she never needed to hide with paint or powder.

Both my grandmother and great-grandmother cultivated herb gardens. And both knew how to use herbs as well as oils, juices, teas, milk, even eggs, in ways that did the most for their hair, skin, and eyes. This art, which women carefully handed down from generation to generation—an art sensible and practical—has been lost to modern technology. But it can be relearned.

Herb gardens can be grown successfully on windowsills. If you don't have a green thumb, herbs are easily available in most health-food stores. The ingredients you buy to make your own cosmetics are fresh today and used today, with no need for chemical preservatives. And you can make as much or as little as you choose, with an added advantage: you can store them in the refrigerator.

Making your own beauty aids may involve a little extra time but much less expense, and the results will make the work worthwhile. You can develop a peaches-and-cream complexion by using—peaches and cream. When you mix an egg mask or an egg shampoo, you will be getting the benefits of the protein from an egg, not a concoction of synthetics. Even oranges can help remove blemishes and soften your skin. And what a delightful perfume is given off by a fresh-peeled orange!

As reigning queen of the Broadway musical theater in the early 1900s, Anna Held was renowned for her figure and for her fantastic complexion. Men flocked to her side—and women were profoundly envious. When she said her sensational skin was the result of bathing as often as possible in a tub filled with milk, she created a bonanza for the dairy industry. Thousands, possibly tens of thousands, of women the world over followed her example, hoping to achieve the same stunning results.

Anna Held was indeed a fortunate lady if bathing in milk was all she needed to keep her so lovely. There are no reports confirming or denying, but I have a strong suspicion she was also careful about diet and nutrition, and *drank* a good deal of milk as well as bathed in it. Milk contains proteins, vitamins, and fats that can perform beauteous feats when given a chance to nourish skin from the inside out. So can many other foods.

The point is, diet is not just a matter of weight loss. Many fad diets and crash diets may take off weight, but at what risk to health and beauty?

Diet, simply, is what you eat. The body requires balanced nutrition—foods that supply it with the proteins, vitamins, and minerals that nourish and feed it in the right proportions. And, of course, we must not overlook the *natural* carbohydrates and proper fats.

Your hair, for example, is composed almost entirely of protein, and protein is the basis of the body's cell structure. These cells are constantly undergoing change and renewal. If your diet contains an insufficient amount of protein, these cells cannot reproduce—they will wear out and die. Without proper nourishment from the inside as well, all the shampoos and treatments you give your hair will be to no avail.

If you are prematurely gray, the cause could be heredity or any number of factors that are out of your control. But it is also possible that your hair is losing its color because of vitamin deficiencies. By the same token, poor nutrition can be responsible for your dry skin, the crow's feet creeping in around the corners of your eyes, and the lines forming around your mouth.

Are you beginning to get the picture?

Beautiful skin, lovely hair, that all-around youthful appearance are not attained by concentrating only on the outer you. Beauty combines good care of your skin, hair, and eyes with general good health.

When you look good and feel good, the world looks good to you. Natural cosmetics, which can be easy on the budget, combined with the right diet, can make this the best year of your beauty life—and next year—and every year thereafter.

The sorry fact is that all too many of us are notoriously lax about nutrition. A prime example is the unwarranted amount of sugar people in western countries consume—about 120 pounds per person per year. Much of this sugar, along with additives and preservatives, is contained in prepackaged foods, the coating on breakfast cereals, in desserts, and even in those popular dried soups. As if that weren't enough, we add more sugar to fruits and cereals. We pour it into everything we drink. And this is a substance that literally poisons the body!

An excess of sugar could be a contributing factor in ailments that affect your beauty potential. You can't possibly look beautiful if you are afflicted with dermatitis (an inflammation of the skin). And that bright smile which lights up your face now will certainly detract from your looks if it shows decaying teeth.

It's time you did something for yourself. Adventure into the "laboratory" of nature's beauty aids. It's a safe, sensible, and beautifying experience.

Chapter IV

THERE'S A COSMETICS SHOP IN YOUR KITCHEN

Following are three reasons why many beauty-conscious women will not care to follow the simple, yet helpful advice in this chapter:

1. They are content to spend money on commercial cosmetics that make grandiose claims for youth and beauty, with only questionable results.
2. They don't object to seeing over half of their cosmetics' dollar go for advertising and another 15 to 20 percent for packaging.
3. They don't mind subjecting their hair, their eyes, their face, and the rest of their physique to potentially dangerous additives that often cause skin irritations, scarring, even damage to the body's chemical balance.

But *you* care about revitalizing your looks, health, youthfulness, and sex appeal. *You* are not content to take risks. It is for *you* that this chapter was written. And for millions more like you!

For you are now ready to discover how natural beauty aids made from staples in your kitchen—staples you think of only as food—can be beneficial from the outside as well as the inside.

Consider, for example, honey. Pure, unadulterated, unglamorous honey. The honey you use in much of your cooking is one of nature's best known moisturizers and facial aids.

Its high vitamin content has given honey a reputation as a skin purifier and nourisher because of its natural acid balance. As a cosmetic, it is unbeatable because it doesn't spoil or turn rancid.

While taking inventory of your kitchen-cosmetic supply, why not try a Honey Toner? This "cosmetic" requires little preparation.

Pat the honey briskly over your face and neck; leave it on for about ten minutes while you relax. Then pat briskly once more before rinsing with warm water. That's all there is to it. A few treatments will leave your skin with a softer feel and a more youthful appearance.

If you don't have a jar of honey handy, as a first experiment try a Citrus Pick-Me-Up, which you can keep ready in the refrigerator. Mix equal parts of citrus juice (preferably lemon) with water, add an extra dash of juice, and put it in a freezer tray. Anytime you feel like relaxing between chores, rub a citrus cube gently over your face. The result will be a cool, fresh tingle, especially helpful for an oily skin.

That's because citrus fruits are astringents—especially lemon, which has been used for centuries as a freckle bleach.

If you're a yogurt eater, you have a simple facial close at hand. Pat the yogurt on your face and leave it on for at least twenty minutes. Rinse it off with lots of warm water. For an extra astringent effect, wipe off the excess with cucumber slices. A light application of safflower or sesame oil provides an excellent moisturizer.

You will be surprised at how many other natural beauty aids are on your kitchen shelves or in the refrigerator. They are every bit as effective as commercial cosmetics, plus far safer and less expensive.

For instance, there is no need to buy commercially made astringents if you use vinegar in your salads. Apple cider vinegar, especially, is good for softening and cleansing all types of skin. It is also a fine old standby for alleviating sunburn. And one tablespoonful added to four ounces of water makes a soothing astringent lotion.

Teas, especially the herbal variety, are also excellent astringents. Add chamomile tea to your shopping list—it has been known for its medicinal values for over 2,500 years. Azuline, an oil in chamomile, is an anti-irritant and reduces swelling—which is why *used* chamomile tea bags are soothing and relaxing to tired, irritated eyes.

If you are troubled by large pores, breakfast oatmeal can be more beneficial than the highest-priced "remedy." A facial mask made with oatmeal will tighten the skin while soothing and healing itching. Oatmeal also makes an effective treatment for eczema and dry skin.

Bran or wheat germ, which should be sitting next to the oatmeal on your shelf, also tightens pores and combats dryness. Mix raw bran or wheat germ with enough milk to make an easily handled paste. Apply to your face, let it dry; allow to remain for an additional 10 to 15 minutes. Remove with warm water.

Worried about unsightly dry or aging skin? Don't look to commercial cosmetics for help. Look instead in the refrigerator for an egg. The lecithin in egg yolks has a softening effect on all animal tissue, and thus helps to smooth skin. The albumin in egg whites contains essential amino acids important for skin health.

For an exhilarating facial, beat two raw eggs, then paint them onto the face with a cotton ball. Allow to dry until the face feels stiff, then rinse well with warm water, followed by a final wiping with cucumber slices.

Cucumbers, by themselves, are also excellent skin smootheners because they contain the softening enzyme *erepsin.* And cucumber juice helps prevent splitting fingernails and falling hair.

Troubled with wispy, fly-away hair? Wine vinegar is not only good on salads; when used as an after-shampoo rinse it adds bounce, body, and shimmering highlights to your hair. Add one tablespoonful to a glass of water: *red* wine vinegar for brunettes, *white* wine vinegar for blond or gray hair.

Besides citrus products, pears and strawberries rank high on the list of cosmetically inclined fruits because of their astringency. So do melons, like cantaloupe, honeydew, and watermelon.

Herbs, usually thought of as seasonings for food or considered only for their fragrance, like lavender and rosemary, are also sources of natural-beauty preparations.

Bathing with chamomile relieves fatigue. Marjoram and mint in the bath water help alleviate nervousness.

One of Cleopatra's beauty-bath recipes was a combination of rosemary, mint, lemons, and oranges. Ninon de Lenclos's secret was rumored to be a bath containing rosemary, lavender, and mint.

Peppermint leaves make a super steam facial that rivals anything you can get in an expensive beauty salon. Steep a handful of peppermint leaves in boiling water and lean over the bowl for three or four minutes with a towel draped over your head. You'll find this a wonderful way to cleanse and stimulate your skin.

Dried or fresh rosemary leaves make an excellent rinse that will add body to dark hair. Mix a handful of leaves with boiling water and let it steep while you shampoo your hair. Finish with the strained mixture as the final rinse.

Most of these herbs are available at health-food stores. Or, to add to the fun of making your own cosmetics, you might try growing herbs on your windowsills.

Lavender makes a lovely house plant. All it needs is a dry and sunny spot to grow in. Peppermint and spearmint thrive in medium-warm temperatures, in filtered sunlight. If you can get a cutting from someone who has a plant, that will trim your cost further. Cuttings will root rapidly in a glass of water. But plants or seedlings are available at most nurseries.

If you start an herb garden, be sure to include marjoram. Its delightful, pungent smell resembles oregano. Marjoram can be grown easily from seeds.

Rosemary is another windowsill favorite. Its leaves, incidentally, are more fragrant than the flowers and give off a warm pine scent.

Making your own beauty aids won't require the purchase of extra equipment. Any of the pots, pans, and mixing bowls you use in your everyday cooking will do the job. Or use wide-mouthed jars instead of mixing bowls.

Try to keep to the suggested measurements. Remember, these are natural cosmetics found in your kitchen. There are no chemical preservatives going into these beauty aids. To avoid rancidity, store in the refrigerator, as some may not keep very well. Cucumber juice, for instance, is very perishable; make it fresh each day.

If you do store cosmetic leftovers in the refrigerator, be sure to label the jar. After all, you wouldn't want your husband drinking the yogurt/avocado face mask. It might be a little too rich for his digestion!

To get the feel of a recipe that requires careful measuring, here's one for a fragrant lotion to cool you and refresh your spirits on a hot summer day.

You will need 2 ounces (¼ cup) of each of the

following: cucumber juice, milk, very strong tea, and witch hazel. Mash or grind a cucumber, skin and all. Strain the juice and mix with the milk. Add the tea next; witch hazel last. Stir in all ingredients slowly to keep the milk from curdling. Smooth the lotion all over your body and relax.

Later chapters will tell how to use the foods in your kitchen, alone or in combination, to enhance your skin, hair, hands—and your sex appeal—as each is discussed.

But, always remember, care of the outer you is not the only essential for beauty. That marvelous piece of machinery, your body, and the skin that covers it, also require not just an *adequate* diet, but the *right* diet for beauty, health, and vitality. The proper combination—super-nutrition plus care with suitable beauty products—is the secret of flawless silken skin, luxuriant hair, clear bright eyes, and a more youthful appearance.

As you read on, you'll discover how to make and use natural cosmetics and, to insure long-lasting results, how to eat your way to skin beauty.

Chapter V

EAT TO GROW A MORE BEAUTIFUL SKIN

"He doesn't look at me in the same old way."

"I used to love the feel of his hands caressing my skin. Now, he seems to avoid touching me."

"Oh, yes, we still make love. But the sight of my bare body doesn't arouse him the way it once did."

How often I have heard these laments from women still young, still attractive. Perhaps, if you are one of them, your story goes something like this:

The early years of your marriage were filled with romance. Affection was not confined to bedtime. Even when you were fully dressed, your husband loved to hold you and sample your softness—with his cheek against your face, with his hand exploring your arms, your neck, your shoulders.

In those days, there was a suppleness to your skin. Your flesh quivered to his touch, imparting excitement to his sliding fingers. Warm, lubricating moisture seemed to ooze from your pores, exuding a wholesome fragrance.

And, oh, the thrill of undressing before him! How his eyes danced—not only at the sight of your sexuality, but also at your glistening back and belly, at your downy thighs and taut calves, unblemished by the so-called ravages of aging.

Then slowly, subtly, things began to change. No longer would your man reach for you eagerly. No longer would he gaze enchantedly at your naked figure. No longer was the sex act followed by cuddling and caressing.

You began seeing some of the reasons in the mirror. Instead of a face soft and scintillating, you gazed at skin that was parched, perhaps even flaky. Where your chest and belly were once smooth and firm, small folds had formed and the flesh was starting to droop. And you didn't have to look closely to spot tiny veins popping on your arms and legs.

So now you're on a cosmetics kick, investing in the finest cleansers and moisturizers, containing only natural ingredients. They help somewhat—but in no way are you able to recapture your youthful radiance.

Are you aware that at this very moment your skin—about fifteen square feet of it—is in the process of rejuvenating itself? Do you know that your skin is an organ—as much an organ as the heart or lungs—and like all organs, it thrives on good nutrition? Can you conceive that your skin's beauty is related to its healthy functioning?

Most of all, do you realize that your skin is your most cooperative organ? If you treat it right, skin responds rapdily—often within a week or two. Let's see how.

But before you read any further, throw away that box of chocolates at your elbow, that oversweet soft drink you've been sipping. Add the pretzels, potato chips, popcorn, and the rest of the usual snacks to the scrap pile too.

Face the facts now. To help your skin achieve its potential beauty, you will have to make some sacrifices.

No! No! Don't draw the living room drapes and get out the black candles. The only magic involved with these sacrifices is the magic you feel in your soul, which says: *you can be beautiful.*

All that's involved is determination and a simple incantation so easily memorized. It goes like this: *"I will not eat candy, greasy foods, white sugar, refined flour, or rich desserts."*

Practice saying it and obeying it and you will be off to a good start in learning what you *shouldn't* eat if you want beautiful skin.

I know, sandwiches are easy to prepare; a hot dog and cola drink make a fast lunch when you're in a hurry. And when you finally sit down to dinner, how can you resist a delightfully rich dessert?

If you want beautiful skin, you will *learn* to resist. These are the "sacrifices" I mean: you will learn to resist because nothing robs the skin of its beauty as fast and as devastatingly as bad eating habits. And bad eating habits are what most people have to un-learn.

Beautiful skin is healthy skin, and the health of your skin is intimately involved with the nutrition of your whole body. No matter how well you apply cosmetics, it is almost impossible to become more beautiful, or stay that way for long, on a diet of overprocessed foods and empty calories.

What you eat determines to a great extent whether you will be leathery-skinned and wrinkled or keep an unlined face and luminous complexion through the years. The wrong diet can cause excessive oiliness and blemishes, dryness, wrinkle lines, and rough, pebbled skin over your face and body.

The right diet, combined with intelligent use of cosmetics, will give your skin a smooth, rose-petal texture, beautiful to the eye, sexually inviting to the touch.

Speaking of touch, humans have the most highly developed sense of touch in the animal kingdom, because our skin has more nerve endings.

As an example, make a circle of your thumb and forefinger and place it over a spot on your arm. In that small area alone, there are approximately four yards of nerves and about 1,300 nerve ends. Imagine what that amounts to when multiplied only in that one arm!

Such exquisite sensitivity is why the entire area of human skin functions as one of the secondary sex organs. From a man's point of view, this is one very good reason for a woman to want soft, sensual, beautiful skin.

But to have it, you must treat your skin with constant kindness, inside and out. For your skin is a hard-working organ. While fighting pollution and germs on the outside, skin is also eliminating poisonous wastes that build up within.

By controlling perspiration, it keeps the body from overheating. It also exudes oils to protect you from tumors, callouses, and rashes. Melanin, a skin component, is the coloring substance that absorbs the sun's dangerous rays before they can harm the body.

Touch any part of you and you have touched an incredible organ that is only 1/20 of an inch thick, yet contains blood vessels, nerves, sweat glands, hair follicles, and billions of cells, all performing functions vital to the body's existence.

The part of the skin visible to the eye is the epidermis. In the bottom layer of the epidermis, cells are continually growing and are pushed to the surface, where they flatten and die. As these cells move, they become dry and tough, forming a protective shield. At the surface, they are constantly worn and rubbed off, to be replaced by new cells pushing their way up.

Next is the dermis, the middle layer. This is basically another protective shield, supporting the epidermis. Here are contained some nerves and blood vessels, lymph cells, sweat glands and the sebaceous glands, which produce oil that lubricates the skin. When sweat and oil are released to the upper surface, they combine to make the skin soft, and resilient. If these glands deteriorate you leave yourself open to dry, itchy, and cracked skin.

Below the other layers, and still in that narrow 1/20 of an inch, is the subcutaneous tissue, the deepest skin layer. In this layer are more nerves, blood vessels, hair roots, sweat glands, and a layer of fat. This fat provides a support layer for the skin above it, acting like a cushion to protect against injury and insulate against cold.

Between the subcutaneous tissue and the body organs is connective tissue, where lymph fluids circulate. And here is where it really gets interesting.

Lymph fluids, constantly in motion, provide nourishment to the body's cell structure and aid in the disposal of cellular wastes. This circulation of lymph fluid keeps tissues alive and healthy. And this free circulation is directly involved with the digestive process.

Notice how everything ties together?

The wrong diet, especially an overabundance of foods containing sugar or starch, can cause a chain of events resulting in skin disorders. Abusing your digestive system overloads the lymph fluid with excess waste, which in turn slows the flow of fluids. This slowdown rapidly affects the condition and appearance of your skin. It can cause bloating and spotting.

The way to avoid it? Eat right!

"But I do eat right," I can hear you saying. "Sure, I have an occasional hot dog, a fancy dessert now and then, maybe a little sugar in my coffee. Is that so bad?"

It's bad enough.

Take this book with you, walk into the kitchen . . . and let's see what you have on the shelves.

First, get rid of white sugar. It has no place in your drinks or in your cooking. The calories in refined sugar are empty; they contain no proteins, no vitamins, no minerals. Sugar forms acid in your system, decays teeth, and destroys important B-vitamins. It robs you of beauty and vitality.

Instead of sugar, buy two jars of honey—one for sweetening and one to use as an external beauty aid. Honey is the number one natural sweetener. It contains vitamins, minerals, and enzymes that aid digestion. It is also an alkalinizer and a quick stimulant. If you miss the ritual of pouring something into your drinks, try date sugar or fruetose, two natural sweeteners rich in nutriments, which you can obtain in health-food stores.

Now that you have eliminated white sugar, toss out cookies, cake mixes, frostings, jams, and jellies. Take the ice cream out of the freezer. Even the finest commercial ice creams are loaded with white sugar and chemicals. If there are children around the house, don't use them as an excuse for keeping ice cream. Give them a break too; start them on the road to healthy skin before they need worry about the problem.

And while it's nice to top off a meal with a tasty dessert, it's even nicer to eat desserts that are nutritionally good for you. Try making desserts using available fresh fruits topped with yogurt, or use the recipes for homemade ice cream and desserts in my book *Cook Right—Live Longer.*

Now, look in the bread box and toss out the white bread and sweet rolls. One hundred percent whole grain bread, with no preservatives, is the thing to buy for sandwiches.

Prepared, processed, and instant cereals go out with the white bread. Use cracked wheat, whole wheat, barley, or millet as healthful substitutes. Remember that incantation you memorized included no white sugar or white flour.

What you should be sure to eat is plenty of protein.

The makeup of the human body is essentially protein. Skin is protein. Hair is protein. Your nails are protein. And protein is an ingredient that must be replenished every day. It's good sense to eat plenty of protein foods for beauty.

Meats, especially organ meats, are the most biologically active of all proteins. Calves' liver, lamb liver, and chicken livers are full of protein. They are also good sources of vitamin A, an essential nutrient for skin beauty. Liver also has from 20 to 30 times more vitamin B-12 than muscle meats. Organ meats are so high in protein, vitamin, and mineral content, at relatively low cost, that you should eat them *at least* twice weekly, and more often when possible.

Seafoods, too, have an abundance of protein, minerals, and vitamins. Additionally, they are rich in polyunsaturated fats (the good kind). Fish is also a splendid source of fluorine and phosphorus, two minerals that prevent unsightly, repelling tooth decay.

By putting more fish in your skin-beauty diet, you will also be benefiting your husband and children or that special man in your life. For the kids will be on their way to stronger teeth and the men to healthier hearts. Among the Japanese, who eat two or three times more fish than meat, the rate of heart attacks for middle-aged men is about one third that of their Western counterparts.

Eggs and low-fat cheese also contain vitamins, minerals and the complete, high-quality protein your skin requires. They should be eaten in some form daily. Now and then, you might even substitute them for lean meat. But avoid jars or packages of processed cheese, as these are artificial foods containing many chemicals and preservatives. Instead buy cottage cheese as choice number one. Also, low-fat hard cheeses that are natural and unprocessed, such as cheddar made with skim milk, feta, goat's-milk, mozzarella, to mention a few.

If you are a salad eater, you are already ahead. Just be sure to mix raw vegetables with leafy greens and you will gain loads of skin nutrients. Chicory greens, lettuce, romaine, endive, and escarole are all sources of vitamins A and C. So are celery, cabbage, carrots, asparagus, and spinach. For something a little different, try dandelion and mustard greens. And for distinctive flavor in salads, top them off with sunflower-seed kernels, which will add B-vitamins and lots more protein. Or try sprinkling wheat germ on any of the foods you eat.

And don't let the word "fat" make you nervous. There are certain fats the body needs. I'm referring, of course, to the polyunsaturates, which help to utilize protein and to retain the natural moisture of your skin. Without proper fat intake, you can't expect to have soft, young-looking skin.

When it comes to eating the right oils and fat, cats seem to be born with an instinctive knowledge of the good it will do them. I am well acquainted with two felines who live with friends of mine. Both cats have lovely fur that shines like satin and feels like velvet. Both of them love oil.

Oil is good for human skin too. But eliminate any solid shortenings, margarine, and lard from your kitchen. For cooking and salads, try safflower oil, which is among the richest in polyunsaturates. Or, in the order of their nutritional value, use sunflower, safflower, sesame, soy, corn, or olive oil.

Eating the right foods is the way to get vitamins that will keep your skin beautiful. Often, however, it just isn't possible to get all the vitamins you need from food alone. That's where the regular use of an all-inclusive vitamin-mineral food supplement can be so beneficial. One of the best formulas, in my opinion, is called Nutri-Time. It is sold in most health-food stores.

Vitamin A is one of the essentials for beautiful skin. But no matter how much you eat of the foods that contain this vitamin, you would have to stuff yourself with them to get enough. And the meager amounts recommended as a routine supplement is hardly enough if you're suffering a deprivation that is harming your skin. Naturally, the amount of deficiency varies from person to person, but I would suggest *no less* than 25,000 units *daily*. If your skin is severely damaged, double or triple that dosage until you notice improvement.

One of the first symptoms of vitamin-A deficiency is excessively dry skin and roughness that begins as gooseflesh on upper arms, shoulders, and thighs. This may be followed by scaliness and abscesses. Peeling, or ridged nails could also be a sign that the diet is lacking in this key vitamin.

When the skin cells are starved for vitamin A, they lose their moisture (a thin mucus secretion in the lower layer that keeps the cells plump and filled out) thus turning dry and shriveled. The pores become clogged with cells that have dried and disintegrated, and the skin becomes rough and susceptible to infections.

Vitamin A helps the body resist all forms of infectious disease—and a body infection, once it develops, will certainly show adverse effects on your skin. So get plenty of vitamin A into you.

The same organ meats that provide the protein you need—liver, kidneys, and sweetbreads—are all loaded with vitamin A. It also abounds in yellow vegetables and fruits ... carrots, yellow squash, yams, apricots, and peaches. And leafy-green vegetables contain carotene, which our bodies convert into vitamin A. The darker green the leafy vegetable, the richer it is in vitamin A.

Vitamin B is a complex of beauty (no pun intended!). An adequate supply can mean the difference between a clear or a blotchy skin. Among the B-vitamins most beneficial to the skin are:

B-1 (Thiamine). This B-vitamin is essential for energy and steady nerves. If you're the victim of a B-1 deficiency, you may have a constant craving for sweets, feel hungry a good deal of the time, be inclined to overeat, have poor circulation, jittery nerves, a lifeless, sallow skin.

Vitamin B-2 (Riboflavin). Extreme oiliness and a tendency to rashes are often an indication of a riboflavin deficiency. A serious lack of this vitamin may show up in coarseness, roughness, fissures, and cracks in the skin and lips. In severe deficiencies, the mouth may become ulcerated. That tiny network of puckered lines around your lips may be caused by a riboflavin deficiency.

Biotin. A serious deficiency of biotin will cause the skin to trade its glow for a grayish pallor, become dry, scale, peel, and develop an unsightly dermatitis. Eat plenty of the B-rich foods to supply you with abundant amounts of biotin to keep your skin glowing.

Niacin. Lack of this nutrient can result in dermatitis, a roughening, reddening, and scaliness of the skin, especially on the arms and neck.

Pantothenic acid. In controlled laboratory experiments with rats, it was revealed that when the animals were starved of pantothenic acid for six or eight weeks, they developed skin eruptions, became old, thin and faded, with loose, wrinkled skin and other symptoms of aging. When pantothenic acid was added to their diet, the aging process was reversed and the wrinkled skin filled out. Dr. Roger Williams, the discoverer of pantothenic acid, called it a veritable "fountain of youth." It is easy to see why.

Folic acid. This B-vitamin, used to control pernicious anemia, is an essential co-worker with your bone marrow to produce the red blood cells that keep your complexion radiant and glowing. A deficiency of it shows in a pale, grayish-hued skin, listlessness, and fatigue.

Liver, brewer's yeast, and wheat germ are among the best sources of the B vitamins. So are beef heart, kidneys, skim milk, soybeans, lima beans, and whole wheat or buckwheat flour. Other important sources: whole-grain breads and cereals, miller's bran, brown rice. Use them all frequently.

Chicken, lobster, and mushrooms contain high quantities of various B-vitamins, as do yogurt, cottage cheese, broccoli, cabbage, and *raw* leafy-green vegetables.

A California model agency advises all its models and potential starlets to add brewer's yeast and wheat germ to their daily diet. Rita LeRoy, head of the agency, says that both these rich sources of B-vitamins help the models gain flawless, photogenic skin.

Wheat germ is great sprinkled over cereals and salads. Brewer's yeast flakes can be mixed into vegetable juices, orange juice, or skim milk. Try creating an original brewer's yeast cocktail in your blender.

Vitamin C is important because a lack of it will show in ugly bruises that result from the slightest touch. Actually, such bruises are caused by the breaking of the thin fragile capillaries under the skin.

By strengthening and firming skin cells and tissues, vitamin C aids in the prevention of tiny broken veins that appear on the cheeks and around the nose—those marks that make people think you are a heavy drinker even if you don't touch a drop. Some nutritionists believe that vitamin C helps in dissolving blood clots that lead to varicose veins.

To keep skin firm and youthful, be sure your intake of vitamin C is plentiful so your cells can soak it up. And don't worry about overdosing, for you can never get "too much" vitamin C. Since it is not stored in the body, a fresh supply is needed every day.

Right here, I must issue a warning to those of you who smoke. Cigarettes waste vitamin C, destroying, on average, as much as 250 milligrams of this vital nutrient each time you light up.

It is not my intention to bore you with what you already know about smoking. I will simply say, if you *must* smoke, increase your daily intake of vitamin C.

Tomatoes, strawberries, citrus fruits, green peppers, black currants, cantaloupe, kale, broccoli and cabbage, especially raw, are good foods to eat for more vitamin C. But in addition to foods, it's wise beauty and nutrition insurance to use high-potency vitamin C supplements.

Vitamin D, while scarce in food, is to be found on your skin. Ergosterol, a substance in the oils of your skin, is changed into vitamin D by the sun's ultraviolet rays and is then absorbed very slowly into the skin and the bloodstream.

Without vitamin D, your body will be unable to burn sugar effectively. Fatigue will overtake you, the vitality and energy that spark your personality will run down, and you won't be able to utilize the minerals calcium or phosphorous, which you must have for your nerves. And undernourished nerves, as you well know, can play havoc with your complexion.

Besides its indirect benefit to your skin, vitamin D, in combination with calcium and phosphorus, produces good teeth and strong bone structure and prevents such glamour handicaps as receding chins, buck teeth, and bowlegs.

Since vitamin D is so conspicuous by its absence in the food you eat, it's impossible to depend on getting enough of it from your daily menu. There is a little in egg yolk, whole milk, salmon and tuna, but the only dependable food sources are cod-liver oil and other fish-liver oils.

Because this is the sunshine vitamin, one of your best sources, at no expense, is the sun.

But broiling on the beach is *not* the way to get your vitamin D. A sun worshipper's tan may look healthy, even sexy, for a few months, but the damage done to the skin will begin to show with time. Too much sun devastates the skin by drying out natural oils and moisture, leading to lines and leatheriness. And overexposure can lead to skin cancers.

There is no need to go out of your way to get the benefits of the sun's rays. Most people get enough exposure in their everyday activities to meet vitamin D requirements.

If you work indoors, on balmy days why not enjoy your lunch hour on a sunny bench in the nearest park?

Or take a healthful walk on the sunny side of the street? If you are the outdoor type or a home gardener, you will be getting much of your share of vitamin D while riding your bicycle or pruning the rose bushes. Any lack of vitamin D can be made up through your diet and supplements, *not* by more sunbathing. Not if you want your skin to be soft, lovely, and admired.

Vitamin F is a group of unsaturated fatty acids that are important in keeping your skin moist and youthful. They are known as linoleic, linolenic, and arachidonic acids.

These nutrients combine with the B-vitamins and vitamin A to change dry, withered skin into moist loveliness. Many cases of eczema have been cured by the daily intake of these essential unsaturated fats, and even that unsightly and tenacious skin condition, psoriasis, has been helped by adding to the diet, each day, several tablespoonfuls of the liquid vegetable oils that are the main source of fatty acids.

Get your daily quota of vitamin F by taking at least two or more tablespoonfuls of some of these natural sources of unsaturated fats: safflower, corn, soybean, sunflower seed, and sesame seed oil.

With these basic foods, you will soon be on the road to skin recovery. But before you get started on your new eating habits, you can speed results by helping your body to rid itself of all the bad things it has accumulated. To this end, I suggest a one-day liquid diet of fresh fruit or vegetable juices. It will give your skin a fresh start.

You needn't be a slave to the clock on this diet. Just drink approximately eight glasses of juice during the day, and a cup of herb tea, consommé, bouillon, or a glass of water whenever you feel the yen.

It's best to make your own juice from fresh fruits.

However, if they are not available, be sure the canned or frozen juice you buy has no sugar added.

Any of the following fruit juices will be fine: orange, grapefruit, pineapple, apple, grape, and cranberry. In the vegetable category: tomato, celery, carrot, or sauerkraut.

It's really not hard. By working from the inside—sensibly applying basic nutrition, plus supplements as needed—you *can* have healthy, beautiful skin.

And if at first you find the adjustment difficult, think of that beautiful moment in the not-too-distant future when you again sense that you are being watched as you undress. Think of a man's hands once more craving to explore your supple softness, his arms eager to engulf you as they once did.

Think of the other thousand thrilling moments you will soon recapture, as you eat ... and grow more beautiful.

Chapter VI

THE FIVE STEPS TO A RADIANT COMPLEXION

Because it performs so many vital functions, the skin is the most changeable organ in the human body. In fact, your outer layer is never the same from one second to the next.

As your protective sheath against weather, pollution, infection, and numerous other stresses, skin takes a continual beating. Small wonder that it has a very short life span.

And that is one of the keys to your loveliness. For as dead skin cells lose their strength and resiliency, the body discards them and sends up fresh replacements. This shedding process is constant, unending—your fifteen square feet of skin renews itself every two weeks.

As you mature, the system tends to slow down and your skin tries to make do with its "old sheath" for just a while longer.

This leads to unsightly, flaky, itchy build-up of dry

surface skin. A coordinated cleansing-care program not only removes these bothersome dried-out scaly patches, it improves the overall texture and tone of every square inch of you. So why tolerate a dull complexion if it isn't necessary?

Restore life and luster to that blanket of flesh that encases you. Indeed, you will see a more beautiful woman smiling back at you from the mirror in only three weeks' time.

Start helping your facial skin do a faster, more effective beauty-repair job when resurfacing itself. If you closely follow the five basic steps below, you will be well on the road to a radiant complexion.

FIVE STEPS CLOSER TO A FABULOUS FACE

1. Cleansing
2. Toning (Exfoliating)
3. Stimulating
4. Lubricating
5. Protecting

Each phase of this regular complexion care has a particular function in wrinkle prevention and rejuvenation of "worn" facial skin. If you work to get your face in top shape, you will be rewarded with lovely, smooth skin with a special glow all its own.

But again I must caution you that external care is only part of the total program to keep yourself looking clear, smooth, and youthful. Despite the best outward treatment you give it, your skin will dry and wither rapidly if it isn't properly nourished from within. There is no substitute for the vitamins, minerals, enzymes, and complete protein foods your cells must have to regenerate themselves.

It is never too late or too early to cultivate a beautiful complexion. Whether young or mature, the skin, when properly cared for, has tremendous powers of self-regeneration. Begin now to give it daily nourishment from within and correct cleansing from without.

That is nature's way to a complexion magnetic with radiance.

Another key to lifelong loveliness is the acid mantle of the skin. Your face, especially, is constantly bombarded by destructive bacteria. But bacteria cannot flourish on an acid surface—so the normal acidity of the skin acts as a barrier against infection.

The trouble is, almost all soaps, cleansers, and cosmetics have a high degree of alkalinity. Alkalis can wash away the acid mantle, leaving the skin vulnerable to infection, wrinkles, and other disorders.

Everyone is born with a slightly acidic mantle. This mantle—or covering—must be kept in proper balance to ward off harmful bacteria.

It's especially important for acne sufferers to keep the skin in acid balance to prevent the spread of infection. Yet with the frequent face scrubbings that are traditionally prescribed for acne, usually with medicated or drying alkaline soaps, the skin will surely lose its protective acid barrier at a time when it's most needed.

If that sounds like a paradox, don't be discouraged. There is an increasing number of products, including non-alkaline soaps and shampoos, that will keep your skin and scalp in their normal, slightly acid balance. Look for the label that says *non-alkaline, natural pH balance,* or *pH factor.*

If you studied chemistry, you know that pH (hydrogen potential) refers to the scale of acidity and alkalinity. It's a scale ranging from 1 (acid) to 14 (alkaline). Healthy, normal skin will register a pH between 5.4 and 6.2. If your pH is below 5.4, you have a skin that's too acid and probably ultrasensitive. Above 6.2 is an alkaline skin, which needs balancing treatment to restore its normal degree of acidity.

Many dermatologists question whether or not the skin's pH is important. They maintain that normal acidity is restored naturally within two or three hours after losing it.

How much damage can occur within a few hours? Perhaps none. But if a soiled powder puff or unwashed hands can cause infection—especially when the skin is in a vulnerable alkaline condition—why take chances?

Soaps and other beauty products with a pH balance will keep your skin within normal acid range. If you're not sure about the ones you're now using, you can buy Nitrazine paper at any drugstore and test them. Just rub one of the little Nitrazine yellow testing strips over a bar of wet soap, or dip it into lotions and creams. If the strip stays yellow, the product is within the pH balance. If it turns blue, it's highly alkaline; purple, it's even more so.

STEP 1: CLEANSING
THE CARDINAL RULES FOR PROPER CLEANSING

- Make sure your hands and washcloth are clean.
- Use warm water—hot is very drying.
- Don't use deodorant soaps on your face.
- Select an acid-base soap—alkali-base soaps neutralize the skin's acid mantle.

There is a lot of confusion on the subject of cleansing because so much conflicting advice is floating around. One dermatologist advises "no soap"; another advocates washing with soap and water every chance you get.

Who is right? Well, everything is relative—to your individual skin texture.

You first must decide what type of skin you're dealing with. If you have oily skin, a piece of absorbent typing paper or brown paper bag will show a transparent halo if you press it to your forehead the first thing upon arising.

If you have dry skin, you will have rough, flaky, dry patches that itch. If you're lucky enough to have normal skin, rejoice! Most women, however, have combination skin—dry cheeks, neck, around eyes—with oiliness sprouting up on chin, nose, and forehead. If you fit that bill, you treat the individual sections according to the problem.

Regardless of type, almost all skins can stand at least one soap-and-water washing daily. But if you are the rare soul who has super-sensitive, allergic, excessively dry skin, use one of the imitation soaps—such as Lowila, Basis, or Oilatum.

Any soap to be used on your delicate facial skin should be gentle, non-irritating and non-drying—preferably enriched with natural ingredients and without harsh chemicals.

Not finding others satisfactory, I designed one myself. Called Lelord Kordel's Special Soap, it contains lecithin, yogurt, sesame oil, almond oil, papaya, lanolin, wheat-germ oil, and honey. It is mild, moisturizing, and meant for fragile feminine skin. It is available in health-food stores.

More important than soap, however, is *water*. It lubricates and softens the parched outside "horny" layer of skin. The function of the morning soaping is to wash off the grime and bacteria that has stuck to your moist skin and the night cream you applied the evening before.

The *way* you wash is extremely important. Women with dry skin should wash gently, using their hands. Those with normal complexions (lucky you!) should use a nubby washcloth (a fresh one every day!) using moderate pressure. Those with very oily skin should wash vigorously, using a complexion brush, pad, or mitt. Women with combination skin should wash the oily areas briskly with a washcloth, then cleanse the cheeks, using clean hands.

Some studies have shown that cleansing cream (what used to be called "cold cream") is more effective in removing makeup. So by all means use that in the evening—saving the soap and water for a morning wake-up.

If you don't wish to purchase an over-the-counter cleansing product, here's a remarkably effective skin cleanser that is fast and simple to prepare right in your own kitchen:

Homemade Cleanser

2 parts of hydrolized lanolin (available at drugstores)
6 parts white petrolatum (petroleum jelly or Vaseline)
20 parts rose-water

Melt the two fats, mix them, and allow to cool. Add rose-water. Beat until white and creamy. This formula will not turn rancid.

STEP 2: TONING (Exfoliating)

Do you always feel like you're wearing yesterday's face? You probably are! And it could be the reason why your skin appears aged and drying. You may be able to recapture your youthful, translucent visage by means of exfoliation. This is an easy process that scales away dead, useless tissue your skin works to the surface. It should be your everyday follow-up to soap and water cleansing. The toner recipe mentioned later in this segment is acid based, and helps restore the protective acid mantle to your skin.

Every woman can benefit from the use of toners, skin fresheners, exfoliators. Those with dry skin should stick to the non-astringent variety (soapless, alcohol-free).

Those with oily skin should use the stronger astringents to promote removal of dry, scaly, dead tissue and to help deep-cleanse dirt and blemish-promoting bacteria from the face.

Men are fortunate in one respect: they have beards. And while many males complain about the inconvenience of shaving, few are aware that their razor blades are secret weapons against skin failure. For shaving does more than remove hair from the face. Whether he knows it or not, each time a man shaves he is performing a method of exfoliation.

No, I'm not about to recommend shaving. Exfoliation can be performed in many ways, without your being ripped off, physically or financially.

Most cosmetic counters have an endless selection of "complexion brushes" or "bath and complexion mitts." Ranging from moderate to exorbitant in price, each claims a super-ability to do away with dead skin cells. No doubt they all have some value—but you can save lots of money by using a nubbly washcloth. On normal, healthy skin it does a more-than-adequate job. It is also easier to keep clean and dry.

Some skin problems, however, may require greater friction than washcloths can provide. For such cases, I have found the Buf-Puf to be most effective in removing dried-up cells, dead skin, and other pore-clogging debris. It is available at a moderate price.

The Buf-Puf consists of a non-woven, self-cleaning polyester web. When used with soap, it may help to eliminate horny rough spots, (keratosis), sun warts, and even minor acne growths.

But, whether you choose the Buf-Puf or a simple washcloth, the cardinal rule is to treat your skin with tenderness.

Remember, too, no matter how vigorously you scrub, confine the scrubbing to the *surface* of the skin. Never press down deep or hard enough to damage the skin's underlying supportive tissue, and be especially gentle to the areas around your tenderest features—your lips and eyes.

There are multitudes of skin exfoliators, toners, and fresheners on the market today. All have the same object in mind—that "little bit extra" surface cleaning to improve the tone of your skin by removing any "leftovers," soap film or dried skin scales.

But one of the least expensive, yet one of the best, is an *acid-based follow-up* you can prepare in your kitchen.

Cider Vinegar pH Balancer

1 oz. cider vinegar
7 oz. water

Mix together in a bottle or jar or, even better, a plant sprayer. (An empty spray bottle of the type that window cleaner comes in makes a good substitute—just be sure that it's been thoroughly washed and scalded first). After washing your face, rinse several times and apply or spray on the vinegar solution.

Variation 1: For oily skin, a mixture of half-vinegar

and half-water may be more effective. Scale the proportions up or down, according to the sensitivity of your skin.

Variation 2: Wet a washcloth with the solution and lie down with it over your face. Relax for a few minutes while your skin drinks in the moisture and its protective acid mantle is restored.

Variation 3: The hurry-up method. When you have no solution mixed and no time to lie down, pour one or two tablespoonfuls of vinegar into a washbasin about one fourth full of water and splash it on your face. Apply moisturizer while your face is slightly damp, let dry a few seconds, then blot off the excess with tissue. You're now ready to apply foundation, powder, or whatever makeup you're in the habit of wearing.

Vinegar acts as an astringent, so if your skin is dry, follow any of the acid-balancing treatments with an emollient cream at night or a moisturizer in the daytime. Chose the mildest vinegar-water solution and never use undiluted vinegar.

SOAPLESS EXFOLIATORS (for dry skin)

For the first exfoliant without soap, let's go back in time and choose three ingredients from a medical document of 1500 B.C.—the *Papyrus Ebers.*

Meal, Honey, and Milk Exfoliator

Combine equal parts of cornmeal and honey and add just enough milk to make it a spreadable consistency. The *Papyrus Ebers* recommended "abrading the skin" with the mixture "and anointing the face to make it smooth," and that's just what you do, in either of several ways:

1. Better stand over the washbasin for this method. After cleansing your face, hold a warm, wet washcloth over it for two or three minutes, dipping the cloth into warm water as often as necessary to retain the heat. With the face still damp, spread some of the mixture on the washcloth and scrub your face with it, giving special attention to areas around the nose and chin. Rinse off with tepid water. While it's still damp, anoint the face with safflower, sesame seed, peanut, or other vegetable oil.

2. Substitute oil for milk in the mixture—it may leave your skin so smooth that you can skip the final "anointing." And instead of spreading the mixture on a washcloth (since oil is hard to wash out) take a heaping spoonful on the fingers of each hand and apply to the face with circular and upward strokes.

3. Put a heaping tablespoonful of either the milk or oil mixture on a piece of gauze or cheesecloth. Fasten the ends together with a string, rubber band, or plastic fastener that comes with sandwich or food-storage bags. Moisten your face and the bag with warm water and "wash" with circular and upward strokes. The abrasive texture of the cornmeal and the friction of the gauze combine to provide a gentle but effective exfoliation without irritating the skin.

Variations: Almond meal, though more expensive, may be substituted for cornmeal. So may two types of oatmeal, the raw, edible kind *or* colloidal oatmeal, available in drugstores. In addition to their mild exfoliating qualities, all of them are soothing and beneficial.

FRESH FRUIT EXFOLIANTS

The enzymes in certain fruits are known for their ability to dissolve surface impurities, including dead skin cells. Remember, though, excessive heat destroys enzymes. So to be effective, the fruit must be raw.

Papaya: Fresh papaya contains papain, the strongest of the debris-dissolving enzymes. It should first be tested on a small patch of skin. For just as soap may cause redness and slight irritation to some sensitive skins, so may a packet of fresh papaya.

Papaya Peel Rub

For first users, I recommend using only the papaya skin with a little of the pulp left on it. Rub it gently over the face with just enough pressure for some of the residue to cling to the skin. Leave the light residue on for three minutes, then look in the mirror. If your skin shows no redness, leave on a few minutes longer. Rinse off with warm or tepid water, scrubbing lightly with a clean washcloth. There is a long-standing belief that final rinsing should be done with cold water to close the pores. This is simply not true. Cold water may feel more refreshing—but it does nothing to the pores. Warm water is a better conditioner for the moisturizers or lubricants that you apply after treatment.

Fresh Pineapple Exfoliant

The enzyme bromelin, contained in fresh pineapple, is similar to papain, the papaya enzyme, in its ability to dissolve dead skin cells and other pore-clogging impurities. But as with papaya, first users should start by testing the fruit or juice on a small patch of skin to see if redness or irritation results. Even if it doesn't—and in the majority of cases it won't—most skins will benefit more by *diluting* the treatment rather than using it full strength. Here are two ways of gentling it down.

1. *Fresh Pineapple Juice Facial.* If you have a vegetable-juice extractor, put a fresh, unpeeled, and cubed pineapple through it. Pour ½ cup of the juice into a small bowl, adding ½ cup of warm water.

Take a double thickness of wide gauze, soak it in the warm mixture, and apply to face. Repeat the application several times during a five-minute period, finishing by lightly scrubbing the face with the juice-soaked gauze. Rinse well and apply conditioner.

2. *Fresh Pineapple Scrub.* If you don't have a juice extractor, cut a thick slice of fresh pineapple and wrap it in a double thickness of wide gauze. Dilute the strength slightly by dipping both your face and the gauze-wrapped pineapple in a basin of warm water, then use it as a washcloth, lightly scrubbing your face. Moisten the gauze as needed during about two minutes of gentle scrubbing, dipping it in and out of the water quickly. You just want to tone down the effect of the bromelin, not wash it away. Rinse well.

Warning! Do not go out in the sun for several hours after any home treatment with fresh pineapple, lemon, or lime juice. Sunlight may cause temporary brownish tinges on the skin. To avoid this possibility, it is better to use them only at night.

The exfoliation methods outlined here are safe, most effective, and least costly. However, you alone, aided by a magnifying mirror, are the final judge of what is most suitable for your complexion.

STEP 3: STIMULATING

While you may not be able to exchange your face for an updated model, you can stimulate the old one to five-star perfection with a once-a-week beauty treat.

How? A weekly facial masque—the wonder worker for "worn-out" skin—the treatment that's more of a treat.

Fifteen minutes is such a small portion of your week to donate exclusively to yourself—to rebuild a "complexion gone gray."

A masque application can make the difference between having a clear skin or a radiant, translucent complexion. It can put a lovely non-artificial blush into your cheeks and a sexy twinkle in your eye. It can add an extra sparkle which may have been lacking for so long!

Webster calls a masque a "cosmetic preparation that gives the skin a tingling feel as it dries." But I call it a face-lift because that's just what it does—it lifts out the lifelessness as well as surface dirt and bacteria.

And another bonus: you get a mental lift too! Your spirits can't help but soar when you *see* and *feel* living proof of your efforts paying off in "youthful dividends."

A masque benefits your skin in several ways. Its main purpose is to stimulate circulation to the facial area. This surge of blood helps even out blotchy patches of skin, which in turn improves and perks up your skin shade. It refreshes the cells at the surface, giving them that bit of "oomph" they need to resurface evenly.

Besides this, a masque application helps slough off dead cells (exfoliation), tightens enlarged pores, and opens clogged ones while making the skin softer and smoother. At the same time, your skin will feel cool, tingly, and refreshed. Just like the dictionary definition claims!

You don't have to rush out and buy an expensive preparation to experience this marvel. Treasure hunt through your kitchen. What gold mine awaits? A simple egg! This wholesome protein food is as good *on* you as *in* you. Enrich your skin with vitamin A, iron, and lecithin by smoothing the yolk slowly all over your face and neck except around the eyes where the skin is very thin and delicate.

Then apply the white of the egg in the same manner. Think of the glamorous women before you who used this very beauty secret! You'll feel like a million dollars, and it's costing you next to nothing.

The skin-rejuvenating egg masque—and other, homemade face-lifts—will give you fabulous results, so why spend a fortune hunting for the store-bought variety?

As the masque is drying, lie down and relax with your eyes closed. Think of all the good it is doing for your lackluster skin—emptying pores clogged with debris, rushing stimulating surges of blood to the "front" to ward off harmful bacteria.

If you can, use a slant board or hang your head backwards over the edge of the bed. This will maximize the effect of the blood circulation to your head.

Just rest the facial muscles. Give them a complete rest. Don't talk. If the phone rings, ignore it. This is your time with yourself. Meditate on the marvelous effect this masque will impart to your tired skin.

Relax and let the masque dry until it feels tight (about 10–30 minutes). When your face is drawn taut, it's time to remove by scrubbing gently with a warm face cloth and warm water. Top off the procedure by applying your favorite toner/freshener/exfoliator. *This is most important* in order to close the now-open pores.

Your face will feel younger, healthier, radiant! Almost as if you could send off sparks. You will love the clean, clear sheen of your skin—and you'll probably wonder why you never tried this before!

Masques can be made from many things. Buttermilk alone can accomplish marvels. At the Bircher-Benner Clinic-Spa in Zurich, Switzerland, clients are given a daily milk facial. For an oily skin, skim milk is used; homogenized milk for a normal skin; a dry skin is given a cream facial. (If cream is too rich for your budget, try half-and-half.) Leave on for twenty minutes, or until dry. Rinse with cold water. Or, as some choose, forget about rinsing and apply moisturizer over the still milk-damp face. Then let dry and apply makeup.

Blender-ground oatmeal, slightly moistened, will also give exhilarating results. Some of the fancier recipes follow, but each and every one is guaranteed to animate a stale "buried-in-bacteria" skin. Your complexion, once nearly suffocated from dried tissue accumulation, will really come alive! For a more perfect complexion, "masque" it once a week.

Almond Meal Mask

Mix 3 teaspoonfuls of almond meal with enough dairy cream or yogurt to make a spreadable mixture. Apply to the face, allow to dry. Remove with a warm, wet towel or washcloth. Sponge face with milk.

If you don't have almond meal, cornmeal makes a good substitute. Scrub face with the meal-and-cream mixture. Rinse well. After sponging with milk, allow to dry for its mild tightening effect. Then rinse off. Apply a moisturizer or emollient.

Powdered Milk Mask

2 tablespoonfuls powdered milk (whole or skim)
Hot water to make a thin paste

Mix the two ingredients in a cup or small dish. Spread over face and neck in an even, thin coat. Next, take a sponge (or washcloth) and scrub the paste right into the pores. This increases the blood supply to the skin. Rinse off and apply another coat, leaving it on to dry. This layer is then lightly messaged off with the tips of your fingers—upward and outward.

Mild Papaya Mask
(for sensitive skins)

Papaya Tea Facial. Bring 2 cups of water to a boil and drop in 2 papaya-leaf tea bags. Let simmer a few seconds, remove from fire, cover, and steep for 5 minutes, then remove the tea bags. Allow the tea to cool slightly, but for best results, keep it as hot as you can comfortably bear.

Dip a clean washcloth in the hot tea, wring out loosely, and cover face with the warm, wet cloth. Hold it there until cool. Keep repeating the process for 10 to 15 minutes, reheating the tea, if necessary. Or you can keep the solution in the top of a double boiler over hot (not boiling) water to avoid reheating.

If you don't mind jumping up at intervals to re-dip the cloth, you can lie down or sit in a chair with your head thrown back. When the time you've set for treatment is up, wet the washcloth again in the tea and gently scrub the face. Rinse well. Apply moisturizer and makeup if you're going out; an emollient cream if it's bedtime.

This simple, inexpensive exfoliant not only removes dead skin cells, but when used *once or twice a week* over a period time, it gives most skins a smooth, translucent quality, like that of fine porcelain.

Papaya Concentrate Facial

This bottled concentrate, available in health food stores, is a popular, refreshing beverage. It is also another gentle way of giving a sensitive skin some of the milder benefits of the enzyme papain. Apply it to the face with a pad of cotton and *allow to dry for 10 minutes.* Rinse off with tepid water, followed with the gentle friction of a washcloth.

Papaya-Yogurt-Yeast Mask

Mash two fresh baker's yeast cakes with enough yogurt to make it a creamy consistency. Blend in an equal amount of fresh, smoothly mashed papaya pulp (the meat), mix well, and apply to face. *Leave on 5 to 15 minutes,* depending upon the sensitivity of your skin. Rinse well. Follow with your choice of emollients or smooth-soothers.

The pulling power of baker's yeast, the slight acidity and antibacterial properties of yogurt, and the debris-dissolving factors of fresh papaya combine to clear the skin of dead cells and give fresh, new ones a chance to surface.

Variation: If you want to experiment with mashed fresh papaya, nothing added, try it first around the nose, forehead, and other areas that tend to be oily, and/or pore-clogged. Gradually extend it to the entire face (except for the delicate skin under and around the eyes) as you see its effect on your skin.

Vinegar and Miller's Bran Pack

½ cup unprocessed miller's bran
2 tablespoonfuls cider vinegar

Enough warm water to make a semi-firm consistency

Apply to the face as you would a mudpack—but more carefully, so it won't have the stick-to-the-face quality that mud has. Lie down and relax for 20–30 minutes, preferably with a towel under your head to catch any that may slide off. Remove with clean, warm water. This is best used at bedtime and followed with the application of emollient cream.

Variation: Add 2 or more tablespoonfuls of honey to the mixture, or enough to give it more staying power on the face.

One of the most effective cleansing-exfoliating masques requires no more than a package of sea salt, available in most health-food stores.

Sea-Spray Vapor

First cleanse your face in the usual way, then fill a 2-quart pan about two thirds with water. Bring to a boil, stir in a heaping tablespoonful of sea salt, and remove from the fire to the sink or table. With a towel over your head, make a tent around your face to keep in the steam. Close your eyes and hold your head over the steaming water for several minutes.

Wash your face thoroughly. With the face cleansed and the pores opened, you're now ready for the stimulating, exfoliating treatment that follows:

Sea-Salt Exfoliant

Combine a teaspoonful of sea salt with ½ cup of mineral oil. Massage lightly into the skin. The salt acts as an abrasive while the oil soothes and smoothes the skin, leaving it beautifully soft after the mixture is washed or toweled off.

Recommended use: Once or twice a week, or as needed, depending upon the condition of your skin and whether it's used as a preventive or a remedy.

Variation 1: Sea salt and kelp granules. To give the treatment a gentler type of friction, mix equal parts of sea salt and fine kelp granules (available at health-food stores) with the oil.

Variation 2: A quick and easy treatment uses only sea salt, kelp granules, water, and a cream or liquid water-soluble cleanser. Mix the cleanser and a teaspoonful of the salt-kelp mixture in the palm of your hand. Apply to the face with the customary upward and outward motion.

STEP 4: LUBRICATING
LUBRICATE TO ILLUMINATE YOUR SKIN

Are you committing facial suicide? You are if you aren't using a moisturizer. The secret of maintaining baby-soft, supple skin is keeping it well-oiled—just as you would any other intricate machine. And your skin is part of the most fascinating, most intricate machine of them all—the human body.

Everyone's skin needs oil—inside (polyunsaturates)—and outside (moisturizers). Who wants to look old before their time? While aging is a natural human process, every woman hopes to discover the fountain of youth. It would be nice if it were that simple. But while the search continues for that miraculous skin rejuvenator, you have to contend with available resources.

That leaves you facing an array of emollients (softeners) and moisturizers (sealants) from cosmetic counters—each proclaiming some secret ingredient that is an exclusive all-powerful answer to your dreams.

While you don't have to stick to lubricants with fancy names and elaborate packaging, you *do* have to use a moisturizer if you desire sensuous, supple skin. Dry skin needs all the help it can get. Oily skin needs smaller doses, with shorter duration on the skin. Nevertheless, in all cases, a moisturizing cream or lotion is needed.

Let's clear up a misconception: moisturizers do not add moisture to the skin. They merely put on a protective cover to help retain the skin's own moisture—like covering a swimming pool to prevent the evaporation of water by the sun. Moisturizers, if used in a regular program of complexion care, can add twenty years of "good skin" to your life.

Dr. Albert M. Kilgman of the University of Pennsylvania School of Medicine found that petroleum jelly was the agent that best stopped water loss and retained an even supply of moisture in the outer skin to prevent scaling. Imagine! Inexpensive Vaseline can do the same job as highly touted, often high-priced commercial products! It's even rated above lanolin, which was long purported to be the skin's best moisturizer.

If you feel your skin is not as beautiful as it could be, now is the time to work with it—and not against it.

To achieve and maintain skin that glows *without* shiny makeup, you need an oil-based moisturizer. If Vaseline strikes you as too messy, choose one that lists petrolatum, or petroleum jelly, as an ingredient. Products containing urea in a greaseless cream base are also beneficial. Urea chemically attracts water, thereby preventing its dissipation.

Dr. Joseph Zizmor, a Manhattan dermatologist, claims hydrophilic petrolatum solution, available at low cost from most pharmacies, is the best and perhaps the only moisturizer you may need.

Cleopatra used a combination of sesame and olive oils—but any of the pure vegetable or seed oils are moisturizing. You can use safflower, sunflower, soy, peanut, or even wheat germ oil. Just be sure to remove the excess. You need not drench yourself for the effect! Use clean cotton balls to absorb leftover oiliness. This oil treatment is great for periodic facial tune-ups.

After age 25, there is a decrease in natural oil production in your body and this leads to the drying out that ends up in wrinkles. If all seven pounds of your skin is dry, forego a tub bath every other day; shower instead. Always use lukewarm water (tepid 80°-90°F) and just pat yourself dry. Don't rub and irritate your sensitive skin.

Nowadays we create our own aridity by taking the natural moisture out of our indoor environment through artificial or central heating. This plays havoc with your already dry skin! The body's water allotment evaporates even faster.

Most women living in island nations are testament that humidity brings out the natural bloom in cheeks. Consider the rosy complexions of the Irish, British, and Scandinavians. Or the almost flawless, moist skin of Polynesians and Filipino women. Their skin is not subjected to abnormal dryness. The more moist climate lets the water within, *stay* within. It is not drawn out and dried up.

•You can take a lesson from this: don't deliberately dry out your skin. Avoid harsh sun. Use a humidifier at home. And most important, seal in the water that's left in you with a good emollient moisturizer that leaves a softening film on the skin to protect it. Lubricate daily *now* so you won't have a "tanned hide" look *later* in life.

STEP 5: PROTECTING FACE UP TO MAKEUP

The use of cosmetics is not necessary for healthy glowing skin. But since most women do not have flawless complexions, they use makeup as a cover-up. This is a mistake. You should select your makeup on the basis of its protective ability.

All makeup is occlusive (pore-clogging) to some degree. So the less you use, the better. If you have oily skin, use water-based products. If your cheeks are dry, apply a moisturizer before using an oil-based makeup.

Don't believe all the advertised promises of cosmetic manufacturers. Makeup has its limitations. Properly and skillfully applied, it can create an illusion of fine facial features—tricks that most models employ. Misuse or overapplication of makeup will make you look much older.

Have you ever seen a published photo of a famous international model before and after makeup? You wouldn't believe it's the same person. The gorgeous girl with the dazzling smile is "plain jane" without benefit of the paint pots. So take hope. Certain cosmetics can add the trappings of glamour even if you don't have the basic features to accent in the first place.

But don't expect *miracles*. Makeup will not shrink your nose to button size any more than it will clear up a case of acne.

A moisturizing makeup helps to "waterproof" your skin against dirt, thereby protecting it. And that's what makeup should do—*protect*. A heavy layer of pancake or theatrical makeup is not only out of place today, it prevents your skin from breathing.

A light foundation can add color to an otherwise pale

face. But if you put it on in gobs, it certainly won't enhance your appearance. You're not going to a masquerade, after all. And if it's not blended into the jawline and neck, it can result in a streaky effect that will detract from an otherwise lovely skin.

Color selection can make or break a "finished face." You have to work with your given skin tones. If you are pink or reddish, tone down with beige or ivory shades; if you are yellow or very pale, perk up with pink or peach to neutralize the sallowness. And please consider your wardrobe selection! What you wear affects your skin's appearance. Black, white, and beige drain color, so you should enliven your own coloring for contrast. Don't let your basic black wash *you* out of the picture. You can achieve a stunning look with a bit of experimentation.

Correction makeup can bring out your best and downplay your flaws. Spotlighting the eyes, highlighting the cheek hollows, and filling in dark lines will draw admirers' eyes elsewhere. And you want to be noticed, don't you? Blending into the scenery is for chameleons only.

Beauty cannot be bought in a bottle or jar, but makeup is about the next best thing. True beauty may come from within, but surface beauty can be created with the "miracle" of makeup. The main purpose of makeup should be to protect your skin (if you select with care) with fringe benefits that can help you add a few final accents to your face.

Of course, makeup will never replace a diet of high-protein foods and restricting sugars and starches. But it is an ego booster while you are eating your way to beauty from within.

Since the object of makeup is to enhance your appearance, it doesn't make sense to destroy the effect by encouraging sun damage to your skin.

You can protect your skin further by applying lotions containing PABA (para-aminobenzoic acid) under makeup one hour before you go outside. This allows time for it to bind with the skin.

One final reminder: *always* remove makeup before going to bed. Wash off the day's bacterial accumulation with cleansing cream. If it's too big a shock for your man to see you "without your face on," you'd better begin conditioning him to seeing you in less and less makeup—or you will wind up with such pore-clogged skin that no makeup will enhance its appearance. Once you've murdered the basic moisture in your skin, resurrecting it becomes a very difficult job indeed. Prevention is always easier than cure.

So guard that wealth of water from within and you'll wow them from without (even without makeup!).

Chapter VII

NEW HOPE FOR BLEMISHED SKIN

True or false? Acne only strikes teenagers.

True or false? There is no way to prevent acne.

True or false? Left alone, acne will go away by itself.

If you answered TRUE to any of these questions, score yourself a big fat ZERO.

Perhaps you are one of the rare ones who have never suffered from this ailment. More likely, you're among the majority who have experienced it in some form . . . in which case, you surely must remember how the acne killed your self-confidence, pulled the rug out from under your ego, maybe even turned you into a social dropout.

But soon afterward by some "magical" process the rashes and pimples started to vanish—and before long the girlish glint and smoothness returned. The change seemed to coincide with the building of your breast line and the curving of your waistline. It occurred around the time when you experienced the need to make love and to share your sexuality with a tender, passionate partner.

And you succeeded, because you were beautiful again. Your renewed confidence enabled you to turn on your magnetic charm. You swiftly forgot the psychological pain you once endured.

Count yourself lucky—and think back to those of your friends who didn't escape the ravages of acne so easily. The ones who were left with permanent scars—on their psyches as well as their faces.

Look around you—at women your own age. Notice how some of them wear thick, heavy makeup. What could they be hiding? Acne perhaps?

Finally, take a long, searching look at yourself. Those occasional blackheads or whiteheads—those intermittent crops of pimples: what are they, if not signs of acne?

Acne is a complex, often paradoxical problem that affects, in varying degrees, 90 percent of teenage boys and 80 percent of the girls. Yet, in spite of this high rate among adolescents, a large proportion of acne sufferers includes members from every age group. This has been true throughout history.

Archaeologists were not surprised when they uncovered evidence that King Tutankhamen, the 16-year-old Egyptian pharaoh, suffered from skin eruptions. Much more unusual was a 116-year-old slave, Ephram Dillert, who had a face as pimply as that of any adolescent on the plantation.

There is no "typical" acne patient, even among adolescents. No two cases are exactly alike, and no two persons respond in an identical way to the same type of treatment. The many clinical types range from oiliness, with a few blackheads, to masses of cysts. Prevention or treatment is not the same for all victims of acne.

ANDROGENS AND ACNE

The major cause of acne is the action of androgens, hormones that are produced by males in the testes. Females produce their own androgenic hormones in the adrenal glands, and both sexes may at times produce excessive amounts of them. When this happens, androgens trigger the sebaceous glands of the face, scalp, chest, and back to an overproduction of oil.

That's why most cases of acne begin at puberty, when a sex-hormonal upheaval is going on in the body. Normally, the sebaceous glands send up small, measured amounts of oil, neither too much nor too little—just enough to keep the skin moist and smooth. But during this period, the pores of the skin first collect the overflow of oil, then erupt in blemishes caused by the build-up.

In persons who get acne, the walls of the pores, like the sex glands, become overactive. An abnormal number of skin cells are produced, sloughing off the walls and accumulating in the pores to form plugs that oxidize and then turn dark when exposed to air. Doctors call these tiny, dark-dotted blemishes *comedones*, but we know them as blackheads.

"Visualize the pore of the skin as the opening of a well," says Dr. Peter Pochi, professor of dermatology at Boston University. "At the bottom of the well are the glands that secrete oil which is constantly coming to the surface. In acne, the wall in that well is leaking. It breaks here and there. The oil leaks out through these breaks, and that causes pimples."

Though acne begins with puberty, when androgens are on a rampage, it doesn't end there. Under certain conditions almost everyone can get it. Only eunuchs, who lack male hormones, are completely immune. Without androgens there is no oil build-up and overflow. Without oil, no acne. At least not the moderate-to-severe type that's characterized by excessive oiliness. But there are other types of acne, three of which are of special interest to adults.

STRESS AND SKIN BLEMISHES

One of the most frequent causes of a high androgen level in women is stress. Stress stimulates the adrenal glands, causing the production of excessive amounts of androgenic hormones. This results in the same problem that affects adolescents: an overflow of the oil glands and a sudden outbreak of pimples.

If you're a nervous, high-strung individual, tension builds upon tension and a highly emotional state can raise the androgen level, increase the sebum flow, and cause a sudden outbreak of pimples on an otherwise unblemished skin.

Since avoiding stress isn't compatible with your temperament, and controlling your nerves, either by positive thinking or sheer willpower is impossible, let a combination of vitamin B-complex and lecithin do it for you. By taking these nutrients every day, you will greatly improve the condition of your nerves, your health, and your skin.

Most people are aware of lecithin as a fat emulsifier, but it's much more. Try eating one or two tablespoonfuls of the granules each day, sprinkled on cereal or salad, in meat loaf or stews, or stirred into a glass of low-fat milk or vegetable juice. You'll like the pleasant, nut-like taste. And with lecithin and B-complex added to your daily diet, you might soon see an amazing difference in your disposition. Suddenly you may find you're less high-strung or worrisome. The result could mean a less oily, less blemished skin.

Even temporary stress can cause acne to erupt—especially when combined with lack of rest. A student, cramming for an exam or trying to finish a paper against a deadline, is a prime acne candidate. A divorce in the family or any other emotional upset—at home, in school, at work—are frequent triggers.

Both in teens and adults, the trauma of moving to a new neighborhood or town, a change of job or school, or even a change of climate may produce an acne flare-up, particularly in a nervous individual. When tension is prolonged, other body functions can be disturbed, including those that result in two enemies of a clear skin: faulty elimination and poor circulation.

Never forget that your skin is a mirror of the total condition of your body, your hormonal balance, your emotions, and state of mind. A program of proper nutrition, relaxation, and exercise can help you attain the physical health and mental well-being that keep your hormones in balance—and your skin unmarred.

BIRTH-CONTROL PILLS AND BLEMISHES

Some types of birth-control pills can cause the skin to break out. If you're on the pill and have a flare-up of acne, find out from your doctor what type you're taking. If it's progesterone, he may wish to switch you to estrogen. That's because progesterone is metabolized into an androgen-like substance, which has the same effect as a high androgen level, resulting in skin eruptions.

Many women can take either type of pill with no harmful effect on the skin; others aren't so lucky. Unlike progesterone, estrogen birth-control pills do not cause acne. But they can photosensitize the skin of some women, making it vulnerable to *chloasma,* the dark blotches that appear on the cheeks after exposure to the sun.

Estrogen stimulates an excessive production of melanin, which gives the skin its coloration. On a photosensitive skin, this results in a brownish skin hue, nicknamed "the mask of pregnancy." When the blotches are caused by pregnancy, they go away after birth. But for women with vulnerable skin who are on estrogen pills, the blotches may last for months. Or in some cases, for a lifetime.

The best approach is not to worry about it (remember what stress does) but to watch for any adverse effect of whatever pill you're taking. You may be one of the fortunates who won't have a problem with either progesterone or estrogen. But if you notice side effects with one or the other pill, it is time to talk to your doctor about a change.

ADULT ACNE

One woman in four is afflicted with adult acne, sometimes called "chin acne" because it usually appears on or around the chin. The eruptions are milder than the typical teenage acne and may occur in one or more large, angry-looking red bumps or in a cluster of small blemishes.

There are fewer statistics available on adult male acne, but if the problem seems to be more prevalent in women, an authority on acne gives one of the reasons for it. "A persistent low-grade acne in adult women," says Dr. Albert Kligman, "is presumptively due to cosmetics unless proved otherwise." In recent years, there has been such an increase in adult acne that dermatologists have coined a new term to describe it: *acne cosmetica.*

In his laboratory at the University of Pennsylvania, Dr. Kligman has tested the acne-causing effect of lanolin, white and red petrolatum, olive oil, cocoa butter, and hundreds of other ingredients used in cosmetics. He found that skin cleansers do not cause acne (but if you already have it, avoid creams—stick to soap-and-water cleansing). Lipstick is not responsible for skin eruptions, and neither is rouge, but be sure to use the dry brush-on kind and avoid the creamy or cheek-gloss type if your skin is oily.

The culprits are the oil-base, pore-clogging preparations that are worn on the face throughout the day and/or the night. These include foundation creams and lotions, night creams, moisturizers, and other oil-base products that are left on your face for hours at a time.

Oily-skinned persons with a tendency to clogged pores and skin eruptions should switch to water-base products. Most of the leading cosmetic companies have them, so read the labels, ask the salesperson, or write the company for information. Moisturizers and foundations containing urea are generally recommended by dermatologists, because of urea's non-occlusive non-pore-clogging factors.

If you are already bothered by *acne cosmetica,* then omit the use of all cosmetics except lipstick until the condition is brought under control.

Though information on them is scarce, men can also be victims of *acne cosmetica,* largely because of oily hair-grooming aids and tonics, or simply because of an oily scalp and hair that need more frequent shampooing.

When the Beatles were at the height of their popularity and their long, over-the-forehead hairstyle was being copied by half of the young male population, a type of forehead acne broke out in near-epidemic proportions. It was caused by oily, bacteria-laden hair coming in contact with the skin and was known at that time as "Beatle forehead."

It's vital for men, women, and adolescents with oily hair to shampoo frequently. An oily scalp is a breeding site for bacteria and can be one of the factors that determine whether a case of acne will be mild or severe. For very serious outbreaks, I urge a daily shampoo and change of pillowcases. Even if they're made of permanent-press fabrics, *iron* your pillowcases each day to be sure bacteria that survived the washing will succumb under a hot iron.

But if you do nothing else, you men with oily hair and a skin problem, keep the expensive "greasy kids' stuff" off your hair. Your own natural oils are sufficient for day-to-day grooming.

CLEANSING AND CARE

The cleansing method for oily, acned skin of both sexes and all ages, from adolescents to adults, is basically the same. The difference is not in the *type* of care, but in the *degree.* The younger, oilier skin of a teenager can take more frequent soap-and-water scrubbings, stronger drying and peeling agents than the skin of an adult—especially a woman's. You yourself are the only one who can decide which soap, how much scrubbing, and what drying agents are too harsh for you. Based on their effect on your skin, you will moderate them accordingly.

Soaps. Cold-cream soaps and those containing oils and other enrichments, which may be fine for dry skin, are definitely *not* for the acned skin. Any good non-oily soap is preferable for mild cases, but for long-lasting, stubborn outbreaks anti-acne soap should contain at least two of these four ingredients:

1. *Resorcinol* for its drying and peeling factors, which slough off the surface layer of dead skin cells and help unclog pores. Its drying action also aids in slowing down the flow of oil.
2. *Salicylic Acid* which has the same effect as resorcinol. Both are effective peeling agents.
3. *Alcohol* to act as a disinfectant.
4. *Sulphur* to decrease the activity of the oil glands and at the same time help remove dead skin cells and other pore-clogging debris.

Whatever anti-acne soap you choose, it will be far more effective as part of a regular regime. For example . . .

TWICE-A-DAY CLEANSING PROGRAM
(More or less, depending on your skin)

Wash with comfortably hot water and anti-acne soap (or any non-oily soap), working up a good lather and getting in a few extra scrubs around the nose, chin, and hairline. Rinse well with warm water and pat dry.

Using a cotton pad or ball, apply one of the astringents listed below, or an acid-base follow-up made of 8 parts water to 1 part cider vinegar.

If you use an acne lotion, wait for the astringent to dry, then spread a thin film of lotion over the entire face, not just on the troubled spots.

TWICE-A-WEEK DEEP-PORE CLEANSING

Scrub your face with soap as in your daily treatment. Rinse. Apply a fingertip towel or washcloth, wrung out of hot water, for several minutes, dipping it in the water repeatedly to keep the application hot.

Rinse your face in warm water, blot slightly, and apply one of the masks for acne-troubled skin. Leave on 20 to 30 minutes. Wash off with warm water followed by a splash of cool (not cold) water and dry. Apply an astringent and let dry before applying acne lotion as suggested above.

ACNE ASTRINGENTS

An astringent for acne-troubled skin should tone the skin, remove any oil left on it, have a drying effect, and restore its acid balance. Here are two inexpensive products you can make which fill those requirements and cost only a fraction of what you would pay for commercial astringents.

Acid-Balanced Acne Astringent

½ cup 70% *ethanol* rubbing alcohol
½ cup distilled water
⅛ cup cider vinegar
1 drop extract of mint (optional)

Combine all ingredients, pour into a sterilized bottle with a tight-fitting top, and store in the refrigerator.

Pore-Tightening Astringent

½ cup 70% *ethanol* rubbing alcohol
¼ cup witch hazel
¼ cup rose-water
⅓ teaspoon powdered alum

Mix, bottle, and store in the refrigerator, as above.

SPECIAL MASKS FOR TROUBLED SKIN

Facial masks based on clay or yeast are most beneficial for oily, acned skin. Both absorb the surface oil, stimulate circulation, loosen and remove dead skin cells. Both have a skin-clearing action and temporarily tone and tighten the skin.

Acne Herbal Clay Mask

1 tablespoonful Fuller's earth
1 tablespoonful alcohol
1 tablespoonful double-strength hot sage tea or enough to make a paste

Mix all ingredients to a spreadable consistency. Apply to face and allow to dry 15–25 minutes. Remove with warm water and follow with an astringent.

The Fuller's earth, available at drugstores, absorbs oil, draws impurities from the pores, and stimulates circulation. Sage tea (available in health-food stores) has mild healing properties.

Fuller's Earth–Yogurt–Papaya Mask

1 tablespoonful Fuller's earth
2 tablespoonfuls strong, hot papaya tea
1 tablespoonful yogurt (unflavored)

Soften the Fuller's earth by mixing it with the tea, then blend in yogurt to form a spreadable mixture.

All the masks in this chapter are applied and removed as directed above. And, of course, you know that any mask treatment starts with a clean face.

Brewer's Yeast and Honey Mask

1 tablespoonful powdered brewer's yeast
Enough honey to make a paste

This simple combination has a strong drawing and deep-pore cleansing power, and honey is both healing and a mild disinfectant.

Variation: If you don't have honey, substitute water. It has the same drawing power, minus the healing factor. (Or use part honey, part water.)

Yeast-Mint Mask

1 *fresh* yeast cake
Cold mint tea

Add enough strong mint tea to the yeast cake to make a creamy, spreadable mixture. But don't let the creaminess fool you—this mask is more astringent and has a stronger drawing power than the preceding one. The herb tea is used cold, to bring out the cooling, refreshing properties of the mint.

All these masks have been especially formulated for the oily, blemished skin, using only a few ingredients that are known to benefit the condition. Other types of masks, including those that soften and moisturize a dry skin and tone and stimulate a sluggish one, will be described in a later chapter.

HOME TREATMENT FOR MINOR BLEMISHES

Tannic Acid Healer—Steep two tea bags (use the cheapest kind—it's strongest in tannic acid) in ½ cup of boiling water. Let cool to room temperature. Pat your face for 5 minutes with the wet tea bags, rinse well, and apply your usual follow-up. Repeat three times a week, or until the condition clears up.

Spirits of Camphor—Helen Gurley Brown, glamorous editor of *Cosmopolitan* magazine, keeps a secret weapon in her desk to fight the occasional tension pimple that sometimes crops up when she has deadline jitters. It's a small bottle of spirits of camphor, which she dabs frequently on the offending spot to dry it up. She always takes it with her when she travels.

Even if a pimple is too full-blown to dry up and disappear without a trace, camphor will tone down the redness and swelling and speed up the healing process.

Both camphor and powdered alum are old-fashioned but effective home treatments for large pores. One of my longtime British correspondents tells me that her beauty salon in London uses 5 drops of spirits of camphor to ½ basin of cool water as a rinse to "tone the skin and tighten the pores" of their clients after a facial.

Laundry Soap—Old-fashioned yellow or brown laundry soap has strong disinfectant and peeling properties. For an occasional pimple, just wet a finger, rub it on the soap, and apply the lather to the affected spot, leaving it on to dry. After 15 to 20 minutes rinse it off, and apply again at frequent intervals until the pimple either dries up or comes to a head.

Onion Poultice—Peel and cut an onion into thick slices and steam them until they become transparent. (If you don't have a vegetable steamer, simmer the slices in just enough water to barely cover them.) Let cool slightly, lie down, and place a slice over each pimpled area. Leave on as a poultice for 15 to 20 minutes.

BLACKHEAD REMEDIES

Tomato Mini-Peel—It's snack-time for your skin, and tomatoes are the appetizer.

After washing your face, carefully wash a raw tomato (there may be pesticide residue on its skin) and cut it in quarters. Using a fresh piece for each quarter of your face, rub it gently but thoroughly into the skin, concentrating on those favorite habitations of blackheads, the nose and chin. Leave on for 5 minutes, then wash off with clear water, scrubbing the affected areas lightly with a nubby washcloth.

Tomatoes contain an acid that peels off surface dead skin cells and blackheads that aren't too deeply imbedded.

Tomato and Cornmeal Scrub—This time you don't have to wash the tomato, because you're going to dip it in boiling water so the skin can peel off easily. Chop the peeled tomato finely, and add about an equal amount of cornmeal, or enough to absorb the juice and make a semi-thick mixture. Spoon the mixture onto a square of cheesecloth and fasten the ends with a rubber band, string, or whatever is handy. Dip the bag into hot water and hold it to your face for 4 or 5 minutes, then scrub the entire face with it, saving the most energetic scrubbing for areas with blackheads.

Any grainy-textured substance, such as salt or almond meal, will help rid the skin of blackheads. So will giving yourself a facial sauna once or twice a week and following it with a mask. Keeping your skin scrupulously clean and free of oil is the best thing you can do for blackheads (certainly it's the best preventive) and the methods recommended for oily, blemished skin are designed not only to cleanse your face but to de-grease it.

Scattered among the fruit, vegetable, and grainy cleansers, de-greasers, and peelers are a few with healing properties. The next treatment, which takes practically no time or money, is one of them.

Leprechauns' Clear-Skin Secret—According to Irish lore, this "secret" to clean, clear, and heal a blemished skin came from a leprechaun "somewhere near Galway." All you need is a potato (Irish, of course!), some water, and a knife. Wash the potato—you needn't peel it unless you want to—slice it, mentally divide your face into fourths, and rub a slice of potato over each fourth. Discard each slice after it's used and start the next area with a fresh one. Use any leftover slices to go over the blemished areas again. And *again,* until the slices are all used up.

You'll be surprised how even on a freshly washed face, raw potato has a cleansing and drawing power that can remove grime hidden deep in the pores. In addition, it has gentle healing properties that are of special benefit to a blemished skin.

Lemon De-Blemisher—Freshly sliced lemon is an old folk remedy for blackheads. Just rub it on the blemishes, let dry for about 20 minutes, and rinse. But remember that lemon juice photosensitizes the skin: if you use it in the daytime, stay out of the sun for a few hours.

French Variation—The French have a milder but more sophisticated variation of the above. They mix equal parts of white wine and lemon juice and apply it with cotton balls. And if there's any wine left over, the French know what to do with it!

OVER-THE-COUNTER ACNE TREATMENTS

Millions of dollars are spent each year on non-prescription acne medication. "They're all a waste of money," as many disappointed acne patients have told me. That's because the odds are against you unless you know what to look for in a product.

If you have only a mild case of acne and won't be satisfied until you try an over-the-counter preparation, at least read the labels and be sure you choose one containing the same ingredients that I advised in anti-acne soaps: *salicylic acid, resorcinol,* and *sulphur.* And for best results, buy one made by a pharmaceutical company, not a cosmetics firm.

Cosmetics manufacturers have, at present, no legal definition for "medicated." They can sell you a product for acne and call it medicated only because it contains less oil than their regular line of creams and lotions. Such products may be better for oily skin, but they are *not* acne treatments. What they are is a waste of time and money for the person who needs immediate help for an acne-troubled skin.

ACNE SCARS

Remember when our parents and teachers used to tell us that "an ounce of prevention is worth a pound of cure?"

For the acne patient it takes equal parts of preventive measures and persistence to avoid the disfiguring scars that result from severe cases.

Earlier you read some of the methods of treating acne in its first and second stages, to control it while it's still controllable and to prevent it from reaching the devastating third and fourth stages.

Eliminating acne scars can be a long, expensive, and painful process, and most of the techniques used will make you look much worse for weeks—sometimes months—before you look better. Some of them work more effectively for certain types of skin than they do for others, and not all of them are successful for *everyone.*

There are four grades of acne, two of which seldom if ever cause scarring and two that may and very often do.

Grade 1. This first-stage acne consists only of a slight oiliness, a scattering of blackheads and whiteheads, and a pimple or two.

Grade 2. This is the most common form of teenage acne. The skin is oilier than in grade 1; blemishes are more numerous and conspicuous, extending in some cases to the back and chest. Neither grade 1 nor grade 2 will cause scarring, so at this early stage, treatment to prevent its spread is extremely vital.

Grade 3. If acne isn't controlled in the first stages, there can be real trouble ahead. In grade 3, the oily condition, whiteheads, and blackheads may have grown to disfiguring proportions that include pustules (pus-filled pimples) and cysts (hard, painful lumps under the skin's surface). Scars resulting from this grade of acne will generally be of the "ice pick" type.

Grade 4. The disfigurement has worsened, the flow of oil is excessive, and there are raised, thickened areas on the skin caused by large, overlapping cysts. This is the condition that results in the worst type of scarring—the deep, saucer-shaped scars or the raised, lumpy ones that form ridges on the skin.

If acne is actively treated in its early stages and the treatment kept up until the condition clears, there is little danger that it will develop into the severe grades that result in scarring. If it's neglected, only a skilled dermatologist can undo the damage—at great expense.

The search for an acne cure or controls is an ongoing process, here and in other countries around the world. The latest and most encouraging report, from Sweden, indicates that researchers there may have found it.

Zinc Supplement Tablets—The external application of zinc oxide ointment was once widely used to treat acne, but modern research has shown it to have little or no value. However, zinc supplement tablets, taken orally, may be the breakthrough that skin specialists and their patients have been hoping for.

After a series of comprehensive tests, researchers at Uppsala University in Sweden have found that the tablets, taken regularly, prove surprisingly effective in acne control.

Their experiment involved 64 patients ranging in age from 13 to 25, all of whom had suffered from acne for at least two years and some for more than five. The patients took 30-milligram zinc gluconate tablets regularly after meals for a period of three months. Within 4 weeks, there was a noticeable decrease in the number of whiteheads, blackheads, and pustules. And after 12 weeks, the acne had been reduced by an average of 85 percent.

These researchers don't know why the zinc gluconate tablets are so effective, but they are sure of the results.

Zinc is one of the trace minerals, and small amounts of it are an essential part of the diet. It is estimated that the average diet falls far short of our daily need. The Swedish experiments have demonstrated that persons with acne may also be suffering from zinc deficiency.

With that in mind, I recommended 100 milligrams a day to a client of mine who had a moderately severe case of acne. In less than a month there was a decided improvement in her skin, and when I saw her again eleven weeks later the acne had almost completely cleared up.

This one test case is the only example I have actually seen of the effectiveness of zinc tablets. But add it to the 64 successful experiments in Sweden and it all stacks up to impressive evidence of a safe, easy treatment for blemished skins ... one that isn't painful, won't disfigure you, and doesn't cost much to try.

And finally, almost any skin problem can be helped by following the advice of the Chairman of Dermatology at the University of Pennsylvania School of Medicine: "Maintain a routine of sufficient sleep, a balanced diet, and regular exercise," says Dr. Walter B. Shelley. "A sick skin can often be healed by a body that is healthy and vigorous."

Chapter VIII

THE CLEAR-SKIN, ANTI-ACNE DIET

Dietary treatment of acne has taken some new directions. Many foods, once strictly forbidden, are now considered possible as preventives.

That is why the following "anti-acne" sample menus may contain some happy surprises. If they sound too good to be true, approach the departures with delight rather than dread. And watch how, gradually, your skin will clear up.

BREAKFAST

6 ounces of any of the following unsweetened juices: orange, grapefruit, pineapple, or tomato

1 cup high-protein cereal (including the variety with chopped nuts and fruits

in it, but pass up any that contain coconut) with ½ cup skim milk

1 cup regular or decaffeinated coffee or tea with 1 teaspoon honey

Mid-Morning:

1,200 mg. Lecithin capsule
25,000-unit Vitamin A capsule
500 mg. Vitamin C tablet
3 Nutri-Time Vitamin-Mineral tablets
50 mgs. Zinc Gluconate tablet

LUNCH

Tuna and chopped celery salad

1 thin slice toasted whole-grain bread with natural peanut butter, spread very thin

1 slice pineapple (fresh or canned-in-its-own-juice) with a generous sprinkling of mint, if desired

1 cup of herb tea with a squirt of fresh lemon juice and a teaspoon of honey

DINNER

6 ounces jellied consommé or clear vegetable soup garnished with a slice of lemon

Small steak, broiled or grilled

Medium serving zucchini or other vegetable (raw)

½ cup paper-thin raw mushroom slices
1 cup regular or decaffeinated coffee, preferably black

Before retiring:

1,200 mg. Lecithin capsule
500 mg. Vitamin C tablet
3 Nutri-Time Vitamin-Mineral tablets
50 mg. Zinc Gluconate tablet

SNACKS

Moderate portions of fresh fruit are always good. So are occasional helpings of walnuts, almonds, and sunflower seeds.

Crisp, sweet carrot sticks and crunchy lengths of celery are still high on the nutritional roster. Try using a little dipping sorcery on them and still stay well within the realm of your anti-acne diet. Here are three delicious dips that help to keep your skin clear:

1 Yogurt and coarsely chopped sunflower seeds combine to add a bit of glamour to these plain little sticks.

2 Yogurt folded into an equal amount of peanut butter.

3 Yogurt with drained, crushed pineapple and finely chopped walnuts. Try cucumber or zucchini slices with this dip.

BREADS—All of the whole-grain varieties are allowed, but no white bread. But please observe an "elegant sufficiency" in the bread department. While your skin may not object to generous servings, your contours might show a difference in a very short time.

CEREALS—All whole-grain varieties but especially millet, barley, oats, and brown rice in moderate quantities.

DAIRY FOODS—Cottage cheese, eggs, low-fat hard cheese (made with skim milk), whole or skim milk (not more than one pint per day), and yogurt.

FISH—Almost all varieties are included these days. Even the fatter varieties—salmon, trout, tuna—are now acceptable. The natural fish oils are good for the skin.

FOWL—Chicken, turkey, even duckling, are regarded as anti-acne foods. The preferred methods of cooking are broiling and roasting. But if you must fry, try oven frying.

FRUITS—Apples and pears. All berries—but especially cranberries. The entire melon family, with special emphasis on papaya—eat it in quantity when available. Pineapple and all citrus fruits are recommended daily for acne sufferers.

MEATS—Lean beef is good in modest quantities, as are lamb (trimmed of excess fat) and veal.

NUTS AND OTHER CRUNCHABLES—Almonds, hazel nuts, peanuts, and walnuts in raw or dry-roasted form are helpful. So are toasted soybeans and hulled pumpkin seeds. Sunflower seeds are especially good for the skin; eat them frequently. Sprinkle over fruit, cereals, and salads for extra benefits of "cosmetic nutrition."

OILS—Corn, olive, peanut, safflower, soya, sunflower, and real mayonnaise with any of the following:

VEGETABLES: Almost unlimited—Asparagus, lettuce, broccoli, and all leafy green vegetables except spinach. Carrots, green beans, okra, potatoes, rutabaga, tomatoes, turnips, squash of all varieties, water chestnuts, yams, and zucchini are excellent for the skin.

BEVERAGES—Almost any fruit or vegetable juice is permitted. Additionally, be sure to drink large daily quantities of plain water "flavored," if desired, with a splash of lemon or lime. Also, regular or decaffeinated coffee and tea (especially the herbal varieties).

AVOID THESE SKIN-DAMAGING RASCALS:

Some of the most marvelous foods from a nutritional standpoint are so loaded with *androgens* that for the acne victim to experiment with them is a chancy affair. High on the list, unfortunately, are shellfish and organ meats. These should be avoided until all traces of acne have vanished.

Are you a soft-drink addict? If so, beware. You may be imbibing *bromides* in skin-harming quantities. Most soft drinks are heavy with *brominated* vegetable oil, a substance to be avoided by the person with troubled skin. So do yourself and your complexion an immense favor by sticking to nature's quenchers: water, fresh fruit and vegetable juices.

Avoid mixers or juices laced with so-called "blushing" seasonings. The most common of these are cayenne, chili peppers, and curry powder. Alcoholic beverages are also "blushers." In fact, anything that dilates the blood vessels is bad news for the acne-prone person, and that includes cigarettes.

Chapter IX

HOW TO FIGHT WRINKLES FROM 18 to 80

You stand naked before a full-length mirror and beam with delight. You have good reason to be pleased—even proud—because your figure has remained quite shapely through the years. It's a healthy, sturdy body, able to give and receive pleasure.

But your joy is short-lived, as you move in for a close look at your face. Crow's feet are tracking off the corners of the eyes. Lines are forming around the mouth, along the cheeks. The skin appears to be losing its luster.

"Why?" you ask yourself. Why does the rest of the body stay young while one's face ages? Is it inevitable? Can we halt the process?

It is a mistake to think of wrinkling as a sign of aging. True, age is a contributing factor, but it is possibly the least significant one. Skin specialists insist that wrinkles can be prevented or slowed down, depending on the effort you expend. The sooner you start, the better—because your first wrinkles have been forming practically since birth.

Look closely at the bronzed faces of young athletes or sunbathers and you'll see the fine lines already being etched around the eyes and on the forehead. Dermatologists, like other specialists, don't always agree with each other, but all are concerned when they see the sun-damaged skin of teenagers losing its natural moisture, becoming parched and prematurely lined. Their conclusion is unanimous: *Excessive sunlight is the skin's worst enemy.*

"The sun's rays do more than just dry the skin," says Dr. Isaac Willis, professor of dermatology at Emory University. "They actually break down the supportive (or connective) tissue underneath, causing more wrinkles."

Connective tissue is responsible for the normal resiliency and elasticity of the skin. When excessive sunlight damages this fiber, degenerative changes occur.

The dermis (or lower skin layer) is made up of about 70 percent collagen fibers, a meshwork of connective tissue that gives the outer skin its strength, form, and elasticity. When collagen fibers become dry, brittle, and lose their flexibility, the skin loses its underlying support and begins to sag and wrinkle.

"Most of the visible changes that occur in skin are the result of sunlight," says Dr. John M. Knox, professor of dermatology at Baylor University. *"Areas that are pulled and under stress are the first to show wrinkles; but the wrinkles would not occur except as a result of injury by radiant energy from sunlight."*

Dr. Robert Alan Franklin, an internationally known cosmetic surgeon, put it more bluntly when he stated, "The sun dries out the skin just the way it turns ripe, round plums into wrinkled prunes."

Does this mean that you must avoid sunlight altogether? Hardly. The sun, remember, helps the body to produce vitamin D. Its warming rays also dilate the blood vessels, thereby increasing circulation and bringing more nourishment to the skin's surface.

Still, "too much of a good thing" can be counterproductive. Too much sun causes dehydration. Too much sun speeds the process of scaling and wrinkling. Worst of all, too much sun raises your risk of skin cancer.

But how much is *too* much? There is no pat answer. Any person leading a normal, active life must take some precaution. If work or leisure-time activity keeps you outdoors, you must take extra precaution. If you are fair-skinned, you must certainly increase your protection against sunlight.

Before exposure, always use a sun-screening or sun-blocking lotion or cream. Try to choose one that contains PABA (para-aminobenzoic acid, a B-vitamin). Sun-*blocking* preparations, especially those containing PABA, have proved more efficient than sun *screeners*.

Sesame oil is the best and one of the least expensive vegetable oils, screening out about 30 percent of the sun's ultraviolet rays, compared with about 20 percent for other vegetable oils. It's also an excellent lubricant, readily absorbed by the skin, leaving a moist but non-greasy look. Don't expect baby oil to protect your skin from sunburn. It is often being used by sunbathers, but it contains neither screening nor blocking properties.

Another excellent natural sun screen consists of a mixture of five parts safflower oil to one part quinine. Or do as many Italians do: mix equal parts of olive oil and vinegar. In addition to its cooling qualities, the vinegar helps skin maintain a slightly acid base, which guards against blemishes, infections, and irritants.

If, in spite of all warnings, you're still determined to

get a suntan, make it a light golden one that does a minimal amount of damage, not the deep bronzing that goes below the surface to attack the supportive tissues. And do it gradually, starting with no more than 15 minutes a day during mid-morning or mid-afternoon. Avoid the hours between 11:00 A.M. and 2:00 P.M., when the sun's rays are at their most merciless.

Whether you're exposed to the sun in your own yard, on a sunny beach, or a snowy ski slope, wear sunglasses to protect your eyes and help prevent squint lines. (Make certain the sunglasses you buy are of optical quality; poor sunglasses can cause damage to the eyes.) And don't forget that you can get a burn not only from the direct rays of the sun, but also from the reflection of sun on sand, water, or snow, and from the wind.

MORE ENEMIES OF YOUR SKIN

Smoking. The damage that smoking can do to your heart and lungs has been so widely publicized that everyone is aware of it. But do you also know that heavy smokers age faster and wrinkle earlier than nonsmokers?

You can make a simple comparison by observing the facial habits of smokers in action. Watch how the lips crease into vertical lines with every puff—how the eyes narrow and wrinkle at the corners as the smoke drifts toward them.

Nicotine causes the small blood vessels in the skin to contract and inhibit circulation. You can see the results of this in the dull and slightly yellowed skin or grayish pallor of longtime smokers.

So if you're one of those who think that cigarettes make them appear more sophisticated, more alluring—even more sexual—ask yourself at what price. How much "sophistication" will smoking add, years later, to a face that is parched and lined? How "alluring" are fingers stained with tobacco's telltale yellow? And just how "sexy" is a breath reeking of stale tar and nicotine?

Poor Circulation. Rev up a sluggish circulation to give your skin a youthful glow and help wrinkle-proof it by sending plenty of oxygen-carrying blood zipping along under its surface.

Any physical exercise is good, as long as it gets the blood coursing freely through the veins instead of just trickling along half-heartedly. Some simple, effective circulation boosters that cost nothing are running in place, jumping an imaginary rope (or a real one!), and taking a brisk daily walk.

For extra stimulation to the face, let your fingers do the walking ... not a "stroll," mind you, but a light and lively "dance tempo." To firm a jawline that's grown slack and creased, or a sagging, crepey chin line, use the back of your hand to spank beneath the chin and jaws from ear to ear. For best results, first cleanse the face and neck, then lubricate with vegetable oil or a moisturizer.

Splashing with alternating cold and warm water also gives facial circulation a lift. However, if your skin is thin and sensitive or has broken capillaries, be sure to avoid extremes of hot and cold.

The Pull of Gravity. If you sometimes feel that "old man gravity" is playing tug-of-war not only with your body but with your face and neck muscles, probably you're right. There is evidence that much of the downward droop and sagging of the face and body can be blamed on the force of gravity over the years. Since science hasn't yet come up with a way to change gravity's course, you have to work at reversing its damaging effect.

A slant board is a good investment for this purpose. If

you don't have one, you can improvise. Upend an ironing board and prop it safely against a bed or a sturdy chair that won't slide. Put a pillow on the end near the floor and relax at least 15 minutes once or twice a day with your feet and body higher than your head.

If you don't have an ironing board, your face can still win the fight against gravity. Simply lie across the bed and let your head hang downward over the edge for 10 or 15 minutes, night and morning.

Exaggerated Facial Expressions. When you pull your facial muscles out of shape with exaggerated expressions, you're subjecting them to a form of stress. Raising the eyebrows, frowning, clenching the teeth, squinting, wrinkling the nose or forehead, and pursing the lips are unattractive facial habits. If not corrected, they will cause premature wrinkles.

Unzip those pursed lips, unclench your teeth, and make a conscious effort to relax your entire face. As simple a technique as parting the lips and letting the jaw drop slightly will do it. So will a smile or a yawn.You can't purse your lips or clench your teeth unless your mouth is closed—so every time you feel them tightening, open your mouth, whether it's to smile, talk, or yawn. Do this every time you think of it, until facial relaxation becomes automatic, and you can prevent negative expression lines from getting a face-hold.

Crash Diets. To prevent a flabby skin and muscles, premature wrinkles, a scrawny neck, drooping breasts, and sagging all-of-you, avoid swift dieting.

When your eating program takes weight off in a hurry, it's often so deficient in nutrients that your face and body lose not only fat and fluid, but a sizable amount of muscle mass. Anyone who has ever had this happen can tell you how difficult it is to restore muscle once it's been dieted away or wasted away by illness or lack of use.

Skin doesn't have a chance to adjust to a sudden weight loss. The body is unable to fill in the areas of lost poundage with collagen, elastin, and other supportive tissue that keeps your skin firm and unlined.

Far worse is the pattern of on-again, off-again dieting. The facial tissues of an overweight person are already stretched too much. Weight lost on a crash diet is regained as soon as the former eating pattern is resumed, and soon the whole process of losing and gaining is repeated. Alternately shrinking and stretching, the skin finally loses its elasticity and sags into folds and wrinkles.

By keeping your weight loss at two pounds a week, you can shape up and save your face at the same time.

Drinking. There is evidence that mild drinking, combined with a good diet, can be beneficial. That's because the dilation and relaxation of facial blood vessels bring a smooth glow to the skin.

The key words here are *mild drinking*—no more than one cocktail or glass of wine per day—and *good diet,* which most heavy drinkers don't follow. Look at the skin of an over-imbiber and you'll see the unmistakable signs of early deterioration: lines and pouches under the eyes, a mottled, uneven color, a network of fine red lines, especially on the cheeks and around the nose. These are caused by tiny capillaries that burst from excessive dilation.

If you've ever had too much to drink, you know how dry and parched your mouth is the morning after. Heavy drinking has the same effect on your skin. It leaches water out of the tissues, sometimes to the point of dehydration. When this happens, be sure to drink plenty of liquids (nonalcoholic!) and try some of the external moisture replenishment suggestions that follow.

Loss of Moisture. Water makes up more than 50 percent of the body's weight. Throughout your physique, including the face, are bones, muscles and fat, surrounded by fluid-filled tissue. If you lose any of these fluids, wrinkles appear.

With increasing age, the skin's Natural Moisturizing Factors (NMFs) decrease, along with their ability to attract water and maintain a normal moisture level in the skin. To give your body the inner hydration it needs, to replenish the fluids that fill the tissues and help the skin retain its moisture, drink six to eight glasses of water a day—in *addition* to other liquids you consume.

You may be surprised to discover how this "treatment" alone recaptures the smooth, unblemished gleam that once made your skin a magnet to the men around you.

Another easy, costs-nothing aid consists simply of a wet compress. Place a tepid washcloth over your face and leave it there for about ten minutes. This will help put water into the skin cells and retain youthful softness for two or three hours.

For a long-lasting moisturizer, splash tepid water on your face after it's been washed or cleansed, then smooth a few drops of safflower, sesame seed, or soybean oil over the still-wet skin. You've heard that oil and water don't mix? They don't. What happens is the oil forms a thin film over the water, sealing in the drops of moisture.

Some oils are too heavy for this, but any light-textured vegetable oil works beautifully and is easy to remove. Leave it on for 10 to 20 minutes, or longer if you have time, then remove with tissue. Make this a part of your daily routine; your skin will look and feel so supple you may decide it's the only moisturizer you need. And, unlike some creams and lotion moisturizers, vegetable oil doesn't clog the pores.

Commercial moisturizers are to be used with discretion. Many of them actually absorb moisture from the skin instead of locking it in as the oil-and-water treatment does.

Since the object of any product you use is to retain moisture, it stands to reason that you must also avoid excessive sweating. Perspiration, along with a number of environmental factors, removes precious moisture from the skin, causing it to look parched. In young skins perspiring does help unclog the pores, but older skins can't afford the loss of moisture.

Many top models spray their faces with water before applying moisturizer. They give themselves another fine misting after putting on cosmetics to make the moist, natural look last longer.

Whether they know it or not, these models are following a sound scientific principle: keratin, a horny substance on the top layer of the skin, can only be softened and made pliable with water.

As the cells underneath are pushed up to the outer layers, they undergo many changes. By the time they reach the top layer of the epidermis, they are formed entirely of keratin and are no longer living cells. This process of growth, maturation, and death of skin cells is called *keratinization*.

While the face is wet, a thin layer of oil (in oil form or in moisturizing lotion form) seals that wetness in the keratin, reducing evaporation. Besides preventing excessive loss of moisture, the best moisturizing lotions actually *add* a bit of water. But even these work better when applied on a pre-wetted face.

If you're seeking to save money, one of the most effective moisturizers is plain old-fashioned petroleum jelly. It's an ingredient of all the best moisturizing lotions and night creams; but, by itself, petroleum jelly costs far less.

Here is another pair of inexpensive moisturing secrets. They come from the kitchen and are easy to use:

1. Next time you prepare an avocado, don't discard the peel. After cleansing the face and neck, rub the inside of the peel over them. Leave on for 15 to 20 minutes, then rinse off with warm water followed by a splash of cold.

2. First cleanse the skin, then pour about ¼ cup of milk into a small bowl or cup. Soak a cotton pad in the milk and pat it lightly over the face and neck until the skin is drenched. Let dry and rinse off.

A hundred percent natural, milk makes the skin dewy and soft. It also causes a tightening action that is gentle and harmless.

To fully appreciate the value of moisturizers, think of a pan of water boiling on the stove. To keep the steam (moisture) from escaping, you cover the top of the pan. The same principle operates with a moisturizer that "covers" your skin and keeps bodily "steam" in check.

A personalized plan to prevent loss of moisture must take into consideration your skin type, your age, your life-style, and the climate you live in. The moist, misty climate of England and Ireland is responsible for some of the world's loveliest complexions. In most of the United States cold weather, wind, and central heating combine to dehydrate skin in the winter, while summer takes its toll with too much sun, heat, and air-conditioning. Dehydrated warm air, indoors, can dry up everything in the room including the skin, almost as quickly as outdoor exposure.

A humidity meter (humidistat) is a good idea for checking the amount of moisture in your home environment. Or watch the humidity reading on your TV weather broadcast. When it drops below 60 (some say 40 is still in the not-too-bad range) the loss must be replenished. A humidifier, spraying a fine mist of water into the air, is kind to both your skin and the atmosphere. You can get the same effect by lowering the thermostat and putting tubs of water around your house or apartment.

Nobody I know keeps tubs around the house, and if you were thinking of rushing out and buying some, price the humidifier first. You may find it costs less and adds more to the decor than the tubs.

A bathtub, half-filled with water and left all day or night, will add some moisture to the air. So will a simmering teakettle or a pan of water on the stove. Every radiator should have a water-filled trough on it during the heating season.

House plants add moisture to the room they're in and give off oxygen too. Spraying them with mist circulates moisture better than just sprinkling water on them. And with a spray you can mist a little on your face at the same time.

Piled-up Dead Skin Cells. One of the oldest medical documents, the *Papyrus Ebers,* dating back to about 1500 B.C., recommends "abrading the skin with a mixture of meal, honey and milk, and anointing the face to make it smooth."

You'll see how well that advice has bridged the centuries by comparing it with modern methods of exfoliation or epidermabrasion, the use of milk and honey in cosmetics, and meal and honey in masks and as abrasives.

Exfoliation (the shedding of old skin cells as new ones are formed) is a normal process that goes on all the time, especially during sleep. That's one reason it's important to wash or cleanse the face each morning even though it had a thorough before-bedtime cleansing. There are about 30 layers of epidermis, and each day a new layer is formed. At the same time the new layer is pushing itself upward, the top layer of dead skin cells is ready to be shed.

Have you ever noticed how much younger the lower half of a man's face usually looks than the upper half? He may have creases around his eyes and furrows on his forehead, but shaving every day provides massage and a form of exfoliation that keep his cheeks firm and smooth. Dead skin cells simply don't have a chance to pile up when a razor scrapes them off every day.

No, ladies, I'm not suggesting that you start shaving! But I do want to emphasize the need, especially of older women, for some type of epidermabrasion or exfoliation to help slough off the dead layer of cells and to keep the skin smooth, youthful, and desirable. Cleopatra did it with mud packs from the banks of the Nile; today we use sterile clay packs, available at cosmetics counters.

The normal process of exfoliation is all that's needed for the young, healthy skin. With daily bathing, face washing, and the friction of toweling dry, the dead cells on a young face and body shed easily and naturally, leaving fresh new skin in their place.

The youthful skin has a uniformity of color and texture that is lacking in older skin. The keratinization cycle (birth, maturation, and death of skin cells) takes about 28 days. During this time, the skin surface is being renewed as new skin cells replace the old. At least that's the way it *should* happen, and does, when we're young. But as we grow older, the cycle becomes less dependable. It slows down, not all over or all at once, but in some places, and the skin is not renewed evenly. The result is seen on many older skins in a mottling of color ranging from dark spots to light, while the texture varies from smooth to rough in different areas.

When layers of dead skin cells accumulate on the surface and aren't removed either by natural or induced exfoliation (epidermabrasion), they form a congestive film that "locks in" crepey lines, blemishes, and discolorations. But this doesn't have to happen. You can prevent it by rousting old, worn-out cells by any of several methods which can be done at home and adjusted to your age and individual skin type.

Washing the face with soap and a nubby washcloth, rubbing gently or vigorously, depending upon the sensitivity of your skin, is the most basic exfoliation treatment. More extensive home methods are described in another chapter.

Poor Nutrition. Nothing, to my knowledge, can age you faster and damage your health, looks, and personality so badly as unhealthful food. Overexposure to the sun, that insidious enemy, limits its destruction to the skin and its supportive tissue. Poor nutrition attacks not only the skin but the hair, eyes, nails, bones, and the health of your entire body, mind, and nervous system.

If you have ever seen, as I have, the wizened, wrinkled, old-looking faces of protein-starved children in the undeveloped countries of the world, you would never again risk premature aging and wrinkling by shortchanging yourself on foods high in cell-renewing protein.

The basics of good nutrition have already been detailed. What more can I say except to repeat: eat plenty of the complete protein foods, fresh vegetables, fruits, and low-fat dairy products. When you use bread and cereal, be sure they're whole-grain and not sweetened with sugar. Avoid white sugar, products made with white flour, fried food, and junk food. Don't forget to add two tablespoonfuls of sesame or safflower oil to your daily diet. Have as much raw food as possible—leafy green salads, fresh vegetables, fruits, melons, and berries—they're great skin clarifiers and wrinkle fighters.

Everything you do to keep healthy, happy, and active has an anti-aging effect on your skin and body, and that includes a happy sex life. It's no happenstance that the skin of a woman in love takes on a special glow and radiance. Doctors will tell you that sexual fulfillment is good for your health and dermatologists agree that it's good for the skin.

So whatever your age, no matter how busy and self-sufficient you are, or how involved with your home and children, or with a job and other outside interests, don't rule out romance. Take time for love. It can make you look younger and more beautiful.

Chapter X

THE GENTLE ART OF SAVING FACE

What do you see when you look into your mirror?

Does your face resemble a spider's web with an intricate network of fine lines radiating from the center?

Is your throat ruffled?

Does your chin look like an accordion?

Your mouth droop at its corners?

Your forehead the image of a road map recording every twist and turn?

If *yes*, you need immediate help. If *not*, you need *prevention.*

Prevention is the major factor in halting unnecessary aging at its present plateau . . . to stop your aging clock, so to speak.

It matters not whether you are the "sweet sixteen" type with the satin-smooth skin of a kewpie doll or if you are the "fabulous fortyish" type with a few living lines adding character to your face—the need for prevention applies equally.

It is important that you understand the need for an anti-aging prevention program to help slow down an ever accelerating aging process. Beauty experts subscribe to the old adage, "An ounce of prevention is worth a pound of cure." They know it requires thirty times more effort to erase wrinkles than it does to prevent them.

Are you at war with your face? Are you treating it as an enemy, endlessly punishing it by pushing, pulling, rubbing, and kneading? It's time you called a truce and began treating your skin like the precious friend it is, with gentleness and love. After all, is there anything more important to you than your own skin?

The barbaric notion that treatment must hurt in order to help is obsolete, especially when dealing with the sensitive musculature of the face. When it comes to the face, the rough approach is worse than no treatment at all. Damage done to the delicate fibers of the skin that are *held together* by the body's system of collagens may be irreversible. Therefore immediately resign from brutal tactics and start treating your face gently, with love. It will respond in kind.

First you must survey the problems.

Contrary to what you may have heard, these problems can be both prevented and repaired, naturally, without the aid of the plastic surgeon's scalpel. Instead of the costly face-lift, the effects of which are only temporary anyhow, you can undouble your double chin, firm your sagging throat, and reverse most of those wrinkles, lines, and crow's feet. European women have been doing it for years.

"But how?" you ask.

By exercising the face.

"But I hate exercise," you say.

Well, so do I. But it's the only way to a more youthful face. There's no magic drug that will keep you in shape. Your body needs exercise to stay in top form; so does your face. What's a few minutes out of your day if the result is a more beautiful, more youthful face?

Flabby body muscles are made both firm and supple through regular exercise. Sagging facial muscles can be reconditioned and made as firm and supple as the rest of you. There's absolutely no reason why you should wear an old face mask on a youthful body. After all, you don't want it to seem that your face and body are mismatched and were created at two different times? Do you? Therefore you must keep *all of you* supple, not just hips, thighs, waist. Bear in mind it is muscle that holds up your face. Regular facial exercises will restore youthful tone to your skin, keep it flexible, and even more important, slow down further deterioration as you age.

If any one group should most definitely know the impact of practicing preventative aging techniques . . . it's the many film and TV stars whose faces are, literally, their fortunes.

Almost daily, they must face the harsh, insensitive, merciless, and eversearching eye of the camera that not only reproduces but also greatly magnifies each tiny age line and skin flaw.

So it is little wonder the stars practice aging prevention by doing facial exercises religiously. They consider them to be insurance against future facial deterioration, as well as a cure for existing telltale lines and aging furrows which add unnecessary years to faces.

Frequently television's youngest stars can be seen on talk shows demonstrating the array of facial exercises they regularly perform as a preventive measure. They know that it is easier to avoid the ravages of old age than it is to eradicate them once they appear.

How about learning to do the same?

"Yes, yes. I'd like to," you answer. "But how do I go about it? How do I begin?"

With moderation, is my advice.

Carefully select from the many exercises explained below those which you feel are most suitable to your particular problems, personality, and life-style. Like all forms of exercise, facial exercises must be done consistently in order to work. And we both know you will not be able to perform regularly those exercises which are in conflict with your other habits, life-style, and responsibilities.

Keep this in mind: it is better to do fewer exercises on a regular basis than sporadically surprise neglected facial muscles with a vast array of pushes and pulls. Never make promises, to others or to yourself, which you know you can't keep in the long run. Even if you can only exercise every other day, that is regularity enough for both face and body.

These exercises, which can be performed in a few minutes, should be worked into your daily routine. They should become a part of your life, like brushing your teeth every morning. And these exercises can, once memorized, be performed most anywhere at any time, in a bathtub or while watching TV. Make it a habit to perform one particular exercise each time you are speaking on the telephone and another one while waiting for an elevator.

However, if you know you lack the discipline to follow through on your exercises, don't hurt yourself by continually trying and failing. Instead, ask a neighbor, friend, or co-worker to do them with you. Set a specific time (whether daily or 3 times weekly) when you and your friend can get together for your "aging prevention" exercises. Soon both your friendship and your faces will solidify and bloom.

Be patient, and don't attempt too many exercises too soon. It will take time to undo the ravages produced by years of neglect. Your wrinkles did not form overnight and neither will they disappear in a flash. Only in mythology do folks turn to smooth stone in an instant. If you wish to restore yesteryear's looks, you'll have to exercise patience—along with your muscles.

Initially, do all of your exercises facing a well-illuminated mirror. It's the best way to make certain you are not creasing some parts of your face while working at smoothing out others. You should also use your mirror to become aware of the particular facial grimaces that are the cause of some of the folds and furrows in your face. Each one of us smiles and frowns somewhat differently.

As we age and our skins lose moisture and elasticity, sags and wrinkles develop wherever muscles are overworked in one direction. The skin can no longer "bounce back" as well as it did in our youth. For example, crow's feet develop from squinting, frown lines from frowning.

As to the nose wrinklers among you who think it's a cute habit because when you were five everyone marveled at it, I want you to notice the very *un*cutesy lines your habit is carving around your nose. Also, have you considered the possibility that what's adorable on a baby is somewhat unbecoming on an adult? After all, was not your first burp considered a marvel as well? Think about it. And then make a determined effort to stop it.

By using the mirror and practicing, you can actually teach yourself to change your facial-expression habits. You can cease frowning whenever something boils over and you must learn to relax those scowl, squint, and screwed-up tension muscles.

Whenever possible do your exercises near open windows. You'll feel more energetic breathing fresh air because it is higher in oxygen content. Stale air is high in nitrogen, which makes you drowsy.

Once you've mastered the exercises, try and do some of them with your feet resting higher than your head. You can either invest in a slant board or make one by propping up an old ironing board on a box. Your feet should be 12–15 inches off the floor. This upside-down position increases the circulation of blood, and thereby of nutrients, to your neck and head. It reverses the constant downward pull of gravity that is responsible for much sagging of skin and muscle, and it removes pressure from other bodily muscles and organs.

According to the forever youthful and beautiful Arlene Dahl, "Twenty minutes on a slantboard is equivalent to two hours of sleep. If you do this daily, you'll never need a face-lift."

Always lubricate your skin before you begin. That will moisturize and soften it. You needn't, however, invest in expensive lotions and creams. You can use light vegetable oils such as sesame-seed oil or just dip a finger into the mayonnaise jar and spread a bit of its contents on your neck and face.

For additional benefits you can, with a pin or needle, prick a 400-unit vitamin-E capsule and either directly massage the nourishing oil on your neck and face or mix the contents with another lubricant. In addition to lubricating your skin, the external application of vitamin E has been shown effective in smoothing out lines and wrinkles. Remember to be extra generous around your eyes, since that area has no oil glands of its own. And when applying any substance to your face, especially around the thin, easily damaged skin surrounding the eyes, do so gently, habitually stroking upwards on your skin to counter nature's downward pull of gravity.

Now you are ready to begin. All of the exercises outlined below are simple yet effective. I have modified some of them to help you perform them at home.

These exercises have worked wonders for the patients of a number of specialists in facial surgery, as well as for the clientele of famous beauty experts and skin-care specialists. They have pulled up many a famous sagging cheek, and if practiced regularly, they can work wonders for you too. Just remember to exercise with tender loving care–TLC–all the way.

Exercise for Unwrinkling Foreheads

To smooth out the area from your eyebrows to the hairline, raise your brows and deliberately wrinkle your forehead. Hold for thirty seconds. Then with the palms of your hands overlapping on your forehead, pressure your brows, lightly yet firmly, back into place. Now, keeping up the pressure, try to wrinkle your forehead again. Hold for thirty seconds. Release and rest. Do twice more.

Exercises for Controlling Lines Between Brows

To unfurrow the furrowed area between your eyebrows, do the following:

1. Whenever you feel tension rising in the area between your brows, gently place the cushioned tip of an index finger against the middle of your forehead, concentrate on it, and leave it there till the tension dissipates.

2. Leave the index finger on your forehead and begin concentrating on widening the distance between your brows by using the powers of your mind. "What?" you ask. Just what I said–*concentrate*–on widening the distance. In your mind's eye, visualize your eyebrows

growing farther apart, stretching the skin between your brows in the process. Keep meditating on increasing the distance till you see, in your imagination, the area expand.

As any practitioner of yoga will tell you, it's the repetition of quiet, steady concentration on an object that gets the job done. The most lackadaisical of your muscles will respond.

Now that you understand that mental exercises can produce physical results, try and concentrate on your object once again. Think of the area between your brows and make it grow wider. That was much better. And not just for the face, but for all of you. If only you would stop and concentrate on an object, like increasing the distance between your brows, each time stress and tension strike, you would have a much smoother face. Tension registers on your face as harsh lines around eyes, nose, and mouth.

3. There are seven steps to this next exercise. All seven can be done in less than a minute. The whole routine, which should be done three times during each exercise session, can, once you've mastered it, be performed while boiling an egg or listening to the weather forecast. You'll need a smooth object, such as a small rubber ball.

To prepare your muscles for the performance of the seven steps, do the following as a warm-up of tired muscles. Look in your mirror and, to the count of ten, bring your eyebrows together in smooth, even steps. Again to the count of ten, return your eyebrows to their original position. Always move in even steps, providing your muscles with time to adjust to new positions and avoiding uneven stretches of these muscles. Repeat twice more and relax. Now you are ready to proceed with the seven steps.

• By using the tips of the thumb and the index finger of one hand, press gently on the area between your eyebrows and push your brows as far apart as you comfortably can. Hold. Count to five, and release the pressure without removing your fingers.

• While still holding your eyebrows apart with one hand, take whatever small smooth object you've chosen to use with the other hand and, gently, for a few seconds massage the area between your brows. Use small circular motions.

• Next, stop all action and with the small object press down on the bone between your eyebrows, and as counterpressure resist the push of your hands with that bone. Continue pressing and resisting ten times.

• Remove the object, and with the fingers of both hands, one set on top of the other, again pressure the space between your brows.

• Look in the mirror, and in order to work your muscles in both directions frown at your reflection. Frown ever more fiercely to the count of five.

• Return to normal position in ten even steps.

• Relax, remove your hands, rest a few minutes, and repeat the routine twice more. By working the muscles in both directions you are counteracting the effects of habitual frowning and teaching your muscles anew to bounce back as they used to years ago.

Exercise for Smoothing Eye Areas

If the area around your eyes is no laughing matter, teach yourself the following exercise:

Use your cushiony fingertips to bring your upper and lower eyelids together to a close. You should pressure each lid equally instead of merely pulling the upper lid down to the lower one. It takes some practice but the results are worth it. Now, while still holding eyelids closed, attempt to open your eyes. Remove your fingers, open eyes widely. Relax for a few seconds.

The second part of this exercise is the reverse of the first part. This time by using your fingertips push upon the upper lids and down on the lower ones, gently pressuring them into remaining open. Then with your fingertips still holding the lids open, try and close your eyes. Release, close your eyes naturally, and rest.

For the third part of the exercise, close your eyes naturally, without the aid of your fingers. Then while eyes remain closed, take the index finger of each hand and lay them in a horizontal position on your upper eyelids. (The insides of the index fingers should be the sides touching the lids.) They are the softest parts of your fingers, and unlike the fingernails on the outer side, they cannot bruise the sensitive skin of your eyelids. Now try to open your eyes. Impossible, right? The upper lids are unnaturally heavy, weighted down by your fingers. Give in to the heavy sinking sensation, and then change your mind and fight back by pushing up with your lower lids. Don't give up. Keep pushing. Don't cheat yourself by pushing with the upper lids. The benefit is in the process of trying, not in succeeding. Therefore continue pushing up, up, up . . . all the time with your lower lids. Now remove your fingertips, open and close your eyes a few times, and relax.

For the final phase, select a comfortable place and sit down. Cover your eyes with the palms of your hands and relax. Allow your eyes to roam about the dark cave you've created for each eye with your cupped palm. Idly explore, without straining. Everything is dark. There's nothing to focus on. All is peaceful and loving. You feel at rest, with nothing disturbing you. There are no glaring lights. And there's no pollution bringing tears to your eyes. Everything is misty and subdued. Think of something beautiful; concentrate on it as long as you like.

This last part is the best, especially for anyone pressured at work throughout the day who must then look fresh and be dazzling throughout the evening and late into the night. Even if you do few other exercises, this one should not be ignored. Because when your eyes are weary, the rest of the face droops along. The musculature of your face is interconnected and when one part tires the rest sags as well.

Exercises for Beautifying Nose and Cheek Areas

These two exercises are designed to tone the muscles of the midsection of your face—the nose and cheek areas.

1. Hold the tip of your nose between forefinger and thumb and, while exerting gentle pressure at that point, attempt to wrinkle the rest of the nose, the upper part. Hold for thirty seconds. Release, and repeat a minimum of four times.
2. Without moving other facial muscles, firmly draw your upper lip down over the lower one until the lower lip is completely covered. Hold as long as you can. Release.

Reverse the procedure by firmly drawing the lower lip up and over the upper one, as if attempting to touch the base of your nose. If you feel it pulling all along your cheeks, way back to your ears, you're doing it right. Hold as long as you comfortably can and release.

Exercises for Toning Mouth and Cheek Areas

To help prevent wrinkling of the lip area and to erase the lines that radiate from your mouth to the ears, marring your cheeks, do the following:

1. Slightly open your mouth and try to move both lips and cheeks toward your temples. Hold. Apply a little pressure at the corners of the mouth, as if trying to break the diagonal sweep upwards of the other muscles. Continue moving lips and cheeks closer to your temples. Hold to the count of twenty. Relax, and repeat twice more.

2. Firmly, but not ferociously, grit your teeth and then try to move your jaw back and forth. Don't worry if movement seems slight at first. Just keep at it, pushing and pulling your jaw back and forth a few more times. Stop. Repeat the same procedure but with your fingers pressed against your chin.

3. Keep your mouth closed by lightly pressing around upper and lower lips with the tips of both index fingers and both thumbs. Now push back at your pressing fingers with your lips, by trying to open your mouth. Hold, and release. Relax and repeat. That's all there is to it.

4. This is a case of whistling your troubles away. Just take a deep breath and then gently purse your lips. Hold lips in the pursing position while slowly letting air run out of your mouth. Relax and return lips to normal. If you prefer song to hot air, whistle a favorite tune. Repeat the exercise while applying pressure to the corners of your lips. As a beginner don't whistle longer than thirty seconds. Once facial muscles grow firmer, in approximately three to four weeks, you'll be ready for an operatic aria or a lengthy country ballad.

5. There really is *beauty in words*. The mere utterance of some words helps restore muscle tone around your mouth. Just remember to enunciate these *beauty words* very slowly, clearly, and extravagantly, and you'll be able to talk your way to a more beautiful you. By incorporating these beautifying words into your regular conversations, you'll improve on your looks. At

every opportunity spice your speech with well-pronounced references to such things as cheese and chowder and church and sex. While you're showering, washing dishes, vacuuming, doing the laundry, or out walking the dog, keep enunciating slowly and clearly, pronouncing each letter carefully:

C H U R C H, C H U R C H, C H U R C H . . .
C H E E S E, C H E E S E, C H E E S E . . .
C H O W D E R, C H O W D E R, C H O W D E R . . .
C H E R U B, C H E R U B, C H E R U B . . .

saving the best for last, conclude with S E X, S E X, S E X . . .

Relax and repeat, not too loudly if outdoors, unless you wish company while you exercise.

Because you can lengthen and strengthen the effect of these words by singing them, consider a musical version of this exercise.

Exercises for Firming Chin, Jaw, and Throat

To firm the jawline and the lower chin muscles and to prevent the formation of horizontal lines along your throat, practice these exercises:

1. Picture the thing you most dislike and, presto, stick your tongue out at it as far as the tongue will go. Hold for a few seconds and draw it back. It's wonderful both for exercising your chin and exorcising your pet peeves. But although it may be enjoyable, don't overdo. Ten times per session will suffice at first. Work up to twenty gradually.
2. Lay your hands on your collarbone and, while firmly pressing with both hands, extend your neck as

far as you can in an upward direction. You should feel the skin on your throat stretching to the limit. Hold for thirty seconds, remove your hands, and relax.

Next, cup your jawline with both hands, and push up gently but firmly. Hold for thirty seconds, remove your hands, and relax.

I hope your chin likes its newly found height, because that's where it should stay from now on.

Resolve to hold your head up no matter what. And to avoid regressing to past lows, wear a turtleneck top once a week and see if you can avoid a creased neck front by day's end.

3. For the next exercise, part your mouth slightly and bring your lower lip over the upper one, as if pouting. Hold the pouting position while saying the word "up" at least twenty times. To vary the degree of tension on these muscles work out different rhythmic speech patterns based on "up." For example: try u-u-up, u-u-u-up, up-up-up-up-up, and so on. Opt for those patterns that please you most and seem to cause the firmest sensations around your chin.

4. With lips closed, jut your chin forward. Then slowly, for maximum effect, move your lower jaw only, first to the right, then to the left. Try to keep the muscles in the upper part of your face stationary. Continue moving from side to side for a count of twenty. Stop, give a giant yawn, stretching all the muscles surrounding your mouth, and relax.

Exercise for Improving Circulation Throughout Neck and Head

Wash your face with a natural-bristle complexion brush, a loofah mitt, or a tablespoon of moistened coarse-ground cornmeal. Whichever you select, lightly caress your face with it, using small circular motions, starting beneath your chin and working upwards to the hairline. Rinse well with plain water or a cider vinegar and water mixture. Pat dry.

To make certain that you are not exercising in vain and are doing everything to keep your profile youthful, do your face a big favor by not burying it in a pillow while you sleep. You'll crease and squash it out of shape. Instead, treat your face like the jewel it is and rest it on a small pillow by training yourself to sleep on your back with the pillow fitting the hollow between the lower part of your head and shoulders. If you find you are absolutely unable to fall asleep on your back, sleep on your side, but get rid of any large pillows. Large pillows push your head and face forward, encouraging the development of double chins and lines on the neck.

When used at the side of your head and face, the pillow burrows into your cheeks and presses the wrinkles of the fabric into your skin as you sleep. There are things other than pillows one can cling to at night! And they won't wrinkle you.

Is a variety of aches or pains plaguing you? Do your feet hurt? Do you suffer from recurring headaches? Indeed, wherever the ache, discover its cause and eliminate it by yourself or with the aid of a nutritionally-oriented physician. And don't neglect mental anguish and nervous tension. Pain of all sort marks your face with lines that are difficult to erase.

What are you waiting for now that you know the facts? Begin today—within a month you'll be surprised by the beautiful results that will show on your ever-so-improved face.

Chapter XI

COSMETIC SURGERY: YES OR NO?

(A New Look at Plastic Surgery)

Step right up, lovely lady! The great medicine show is about to begin!

No, it's not snake oil they're selling, but honest-to-goodness treatments endorsed by your family physician and the medical associations. They offer to remove inches from your physique, years from your age—and lots of money from your bank account!

Are you interested? Let's take a look at some average fees.

For a full face-lift, be prepared to invest anywhere from two to five thousand dollars.

A standard "nose job" nowadays costs around two thousand.

Add two thousand more for firming up a weak chin.

Top it off with another thousand for a skin peel.

Depending on how much you're able to afford, you can have one or all of these treatments. Or while there's still time, you can take an alternative: *self-care.* So invest now toward a future more beautiful you.

Currently the fastest-growing medical specialty, the art of plastic surgery is many centuries old. Records show that as long as nine hundrend years ago doctors in India were repairing and even replacing damaged noses. Ancient Chinese physicians were able to fix cleft palates (hair-lips) in much the same manner as today's surgeons.

Originally conceived as a therapeutic technique for persons with health-harming birth defects, plastic surgery rapidly expanded to include damage caused by accidents. And for many a combat soldier, whose features were shattered beyond recognition, plastic surgeons did indeed perform "miraculous" cures.

These successes provided the impetus for a subbranch of this marvelous therapy, called cosmetic surgery. And it is this phase that primarily interests today's beauty-conscious woman.

Before dwelling on the pros and cons of cosmetic surgery, I must point out what it can *not* do for you.

Many a woman enters the surgeon's office with a picture of a movie star or a fashion model, declaring, "I want to look like her." Any reputable surgeon will say forget it—he's not in the business of "changing" faces. Surgeons can only improve upon what already exists.

Another common belief is that face-lifting will change your personality. This too is an exaggeration. True, the youngish look that results from a well-done operation gives the spirits an enormous lift and the ego a tremendous boost. But your plastic surgeon is not a psychiatrist, and his scalpel cannot excise deep-rooted emotional problems.

The most prevalent fallacy of all is the notion that cosmetic surgery produces lifetime results.

Eleanor is a case in point. "A face-lift certainly makes a difference, doesn't it!" she exclaimed when she visited me for nutritional consultation.

Eleanor had recently undergone some extensive (and expensive) surgery. The result was nothing short of sensational. But as Eleanor kept prodding me for compliments, I realized I'd be doing her a disservice if I didn't offer some words of admonition.

"Eleanor," I said, "you look lovely and a good deal younger, but . . ."

"But nothing!" she interrupted. "Now, when I tell people I'm in my thirties, I'm sure they believe me."

"I'm sure they do too. But how long will that last?"

"For the rest of my life, I assume. Oh, I know I won't always look like a mid-thirty-year-old, but at least I'll appear to be ten or fifteen years younger than I really am."

"Eleanor," I warned, "if you just sit around admiring your new look, in a few years you'll be back on the operating table."

"How come?" Eleanor asked, crestfallen.

"Let me put it this way," I replied. "Why did you decide on a face-lift in the first place?"

"Well, it was my sagging jowls and droopy chin that sent me to the plastic surgeon."

"And are you aware that if you'd concentrated on the *cause* of those sagging jowls, Eleanor, you probably could have gone without that face-lift?"

Eleanor's problems, I explained, like most facial problems that lead women down the plastic-surgery path, usually result from lack of tone in the muscles under the skin. Sagging jowls are one symptom of this lack of muscle tone, and a face-lift will correct *only the symptom*.

What the surgeon hasn't gotten at is the cause. That is strictly up to the patient, who has probably been ignoring the cause all her life. If she continues to do so, she can look forward to another expensive face-lift in the not-too-distant future.

Once on that kick, she will eventually need another face-lift, and another, and possibly another. The more operations she has, the tighter her skin will appear and her face may end up looking like a marble mask.

You have seen that marble look among prominent celebrities. A face that doesn't actually appear younger or even beautiful, but seems frozen in time. Too much surgery has taken all the expression from the face so that what it most resembles is a statue, interesting to look at but unreal, unbelievable, even a little frightening.

Unlike statues, human faces most mature to match the passing years. It becomes a woman to look warm and womanly, for regardless of what television and the movies would have you believe, most men prefer women who don't forever look like young girls.

"Oh, must you be the voice of gloom?" Eleanor asked. "What else is a woman to do when her face shows her age?"

"You can postpone the probability of another face-lift indefinitely," I assured her, "by following the same advice I offer to women who've never had their faces worked on."

Many women spend a great deal of time exercising to keep themselves young-looking and attractive. They work diligently at slimming their waists and building their busts. They perform strenuous gyrations to tighten thighs and calves, to de-flab buttocks, to firm their arms.

And that's as it should be. For the woman who wishes to keep bulges from spoiling the size of dresses she's been wearing since age eighteen, an exercise regime is necessary to keep muscles from becoming loose and slack.

Yet these same women, conscientious about their figures from the neck down, completely ignore one of their most vital features—their faces. It is as if they are resigned to wrinkled cheeks and sagging jowls.

Why this sense of hopelessness? Strangely, I've found that too many people are unaware of a simple, obvious fact: the face and neck are as much dependent on muscles as the rest of the body.

Fifty-five of them, to be exact. That's the number of face-and-neck muscles that need constant firming.

Exercise creates strong bodies by increasing blood circulation. To be sure that facial and neck muscles reap the benefits from increased circulation, you must do exercises specifically aimed at strengthening these muscles.

And you must not make the mistake, as many people do, of regarding strenuous sports as face exercisers. It's true that activities like tennis, handball, even golf, cause a lot of frowning, grimacing, and squinting. But that's what I call negative exercise, because it's helping to add lines to your complexion.

The right kind of facial exercise concentrates on tightening muscles to help eliminate lines and sagging. Here are a couple of exercises you might try for starters. It's a good idea to do them in front of a mirror, until you get the hang of them.

JAW JOGGER

Ready? Pretend you are whistling for a dog. Form the whistle ... now hold that position and move your mouth slowly around in a circle, first to one side for a count of five, then to the other side for a count of five. Feel those muscles working? Repeat this exercise as often as you can throughout the day, but be sure to do it at least twice a day.

DOUBLE-CHIN CHASER

Imagine you are the heroine caught at a frightful moment in your favorite horror movie. Open your mouth and eyes wide and scream silently. I mean SCREAM. Hold for a count of five, relax for a minute and scream twice more, each time for a five-count, relaxing between screams.

These exercises bring dozens of muscles into play. While holding the scream, put your hand on your neck under your chin and feel how the muscles tighten. When you do this one in front of a mirror, you will notice that you are also exercising muscles under and around your eyes.

If your face feels warm and tingly, even a trifle stiff after this workout, that's fine. Those are good signs . . . signs that you are making neglected muscles function again.

And don't worry about being caught making faces. Include your man in your exercise program and he won't make fun of you. All of us are concerned about the way we look. When people care about each other, whether it's husband or lover, it can add to their romance by working on their attractiveness together.

Of course, not everyone will need or can afford a complete face-lift. Even among people who never exercise, there are some fortunate few who can remedy their aged appearances by undergoing one of the less complicated, less expensive techniques. In this regard, basic eye surgery is sometimes worth considering.

When eyes don't receive proper exercise or nourishment, fatty tissue starts to deposit under the lower lids.

After a few years puffiness develops—and finally that unsightly condition known as "bags" under the eyes.

This feature can be eliminated through relatively inexpensive under-eye surgery. By removing fatty cells and a little of the muscle, the surgeon is able to soften the bags, causing them to disappear.

For eyes that look droopy or wrinkled because of overhanging lids, upper-eye surgery—or an eye-lift—is frequently recommended. It is the simplest plastic surgery to perform, since the scar left by the incision is concealed in the natural crease of the eyelid. And because it is one of the easiest cosmetic operations, it is also among the most affordable.

But whether or not you can afford surgery, your goal should be to avoid the necessity. To do that, you must begin treating your eyes long before those unsightly symptoms develop. Like right now.

The next two exercises will go a long way toward strengthening under-eye muscles, preventing bags, and erasing wrinkles. So—back to your mirror . . .

EYE UN-LINER

Look into the mirror and squeeze one eye tightly shut. Watch how the under-eye area tightens. Do this alternately with each eye, but do it slowly. Count one-and-two-and-three, then change eyes and repeat the routine five times.

UNDER-EYE FIRMER

Try forcing your eyes to close while you fight the effort by pulling down with your fingers on your cheekbones. Practice in the mirror until you get it. Notice how you are exercising all those small muscles.

These exercises, too, should be performed as often as possible.

Another area requiring constant exercise is the neck—one of the first places to show signs of sagging. You don't want to end up with a firm face and a neck with jowls that droop like a turkey gobbler.

I never cease to be amazed at the number of people who forget how important good posture is to a youthful look. One of the tricks to keeping a youthful neck is to hold it firm and straight when you walk, with head held high.

Practice walking across the room *now*, holding your neck stretched back and up. Think of that alluring head of Nefertiti. When you walk down the street, imagine yourself a princess in a procession. Keep your chin in. Don't walk with head bent and neck crooked.

As other heads turn to look at you, your man will realize just how lovely and attractive you are—and how lucky he is. It will probably make him hold his head and neck straighter and walk like a prince. That's why, whoever he is, you should get your "prince" to work on these exercises with you.

NECK SLIMMERS

To tone neck and chin muscles, sit up straight, lean your head back as far as you can. All set? Now, roll your head in a circle. That's it. Slowly over to one side, now forward, keep rolling to the other side, then to the back again. Think of yourself as a rag doll whose neck has no bones. Try to work up to about five or six neck rolls daily.

Or sit up straight and fold your arms across your waist. Hold your head high. Ready? Bend your head slowly forward and try to touch your chin to your chest. Come up slowly. Try to touch your head to one shoulder. Up slowly. Try to touch the other shoulder with your head. You won't make it, but try. Do these alternately—forward, side, side. Count ... one and up and side and up and side and up. Repeat at least three times.

Keep to these exercises regularly and you will never need to hide your neck with scarves. Indeed, you will carry your neck proudly.

Now that you are well on your way to an alluring neck and a firm chin, take a good look at your mouth. Does it show a pleasant expression or are lines and furrows beginning to form around it?

One way to eliminate droopy mouth lines is to cultivate pleasant thoughts that lead to relaxed facial expressions. Look around you at the solemn and sullen attitudes on so many faces, and the lines that develop and remain, getting deeper and deeper. Smiling often is another way to eliminate those lines.

But to exercise away lines that have already formed, start practicing the following:

THE SMILER

Stand in front of your mirror and smile with your mouth closed. Slowly, slowly, there it goes. Keep your lips together and push that smile as far up on your face as you can, until you really feel the pull. When you look like the grinning clown on a circus poster you are doing it right, and strengthening chin muscles at the same time.

FROWN ERASER

Use the same principle as with the exercise to strengthen under-eye muscles. Try to make those furrows move upward while you exert downward pressure, then try to pull them down while exerting upward pressure. Count to five in each direction.

While embarking on an exercise regime, it is also vital to eliminate certain wrong facial gymnastics. These include the contortions caused by frowning, grimacing, squinting and forehead wrinkling. The lines they cause are often the most difficult to eliminate, because they result from bad habits. Exercise will help—but unless you learn to control the habits, those furrows will never even soften, let alone vanish.

Most important, try to prevent yourself from frowning. How? I know it's easier said than done, but one way is to keep reminding yourself. Whenever you're alone, you might try sticking cellophane tape tightly across your forehead. Every time you frown, the pull of the tape will serve as a reminder, thus helping you to break the habit.

I must caution you, however, that exercise alone will not save you from a trip to the plastic surgeon. For while the object of exercising is to increase blood circulation and spread nutrients through the body, there won't be many benefits showing unless you supply the right nutrients.

And beauty, as I keep stressing, begins with protein.

This is the most important nutrient the body needs to keep muscles from becoming weak. Many professional athletes, while they may not all be beautiful, are always on a high-protein diet because their muscles are their livelihood. With them it is an accepted fact: protein strengthens muscles.

But relax ... I'm not trying to turn you into a lady wrestler or a female fullback! What we are aiming for is strong, firm facial muscles ... muscles that won't sag ... muscles that will save you a visit to a plastic surgeon.

The dermis, our second layer of skin, is made up primarily of collagen, the connective protein that tightens and firms body cells. If your body lacks protein, this is the first place that will show signs of breakdown, leading to sagging and drooping.

A diet of high-protein foods repairs and rebuilds worn-out tissues. It's another form of insurance to keep you young-looking and forestall the need for cosmetic surgery. That's what makes it worth the effort. All it really takes is more attention to what you eat and what you cook. Then you and your man will stay young-looking together.

Think of a high-protein diet as "exercise food." That's not exaggeration, since proteins stimulate body cells into constant exercise—firming, tightening, rebuilding, and repairing themselves.

You can make a start by including liver in your diet. All kinds of liver—calves' liver, chicken liver, beef liver, lamb liver. Liver has more nutritional value than most other foods. So important is liver, in fact, that if you are unable to develop a taste for it, consider using desiccated liver powder or tablets.

A good "anti-surgery diet" must also include eggs, low-fat cheese, lean meat, seafood, and skim milk—all excellent sources of protein.

Keep this fact in mind: no amount of exercise or proper nutrition can eliminate such features as a crooked or overly large nose or outsized ears. Nor would I discourage cosmetic surgery in such instances. If an operation can help rid you of a feeling of ugliness, it is worth the effort and expense for the psychological benefits you'll derive.

But a word of warning: plastic surgeons are never able to guarantee results. No reputable surgeon will even assure you that his operation will make you prettier. That's why nearly all of these specialists request their fees in advance. Too often, they claim, they were "burned" by patients who expected miracles and wound up disillusioned.

For wrinkles or sagging muscles, however, a regular exercise-nutrition regime offers a viable alternative that can forestall face-lifting for a very long time—perhaps forever—while bringing out your true, natural loveliness.

Chapter XII

HEALTHY HAIR: YOUR CROWNING GLORY

It is your most fickle feature. On some days, it totally obeys your wishes, falling into place with the mere stroke of a brush. At other times, it turns ornery, snarling and snagging, refusing to stay put.

Throughout history, it has borne such glamorous labels as *bouffant, gamin* and *chignon*—or the more earthy *shag, pageboy,* and *ponytail*. It has even been named after personalities as diverse as Cleopatra and Madame Pompadour.

Hair ... it can be friend or foe. If you neglect it, hair is quick to respond with brittleness and dullness—enough to mar the most dazzling of beauties. But treat it right and hair will be your partner in lifelong loveliness.

For lustrous hair is your shining symbol of femininity—the frame for that work of art, your face. It is one of your first features to catch a man's eye—indeed, all eyes.

There are myriad ways to keep your hair glowing like a beacon. Some women spend hours teasing or curling, bleaching or tinting, cutting or shaping. Others invest literally hundreds of dollars a month in professional upkeep.

Yet, while your hair deserves to be lavished with loving care, no amount of external treatment will bring out its full, glittering promise unless it is also "beautified" from within. For every hair follicle is rooted firmly in nerves and blood vessels, which feed it with nutrients flowing in your bloodstream.

Although the quality of hair is predetermined by your genes, you can make the most of what you have by fortifying your diet with the foods your follicles need to formulate beautiful, glossy hair:

Protein, the number-one nutriment for glorious hair, which is itself nearly all protein. The best sources are beef, lamb, poultry, fish, liver, heart, kidneys, eggs, low-fat cheese, brewer's yeast, avocado, cornmeal, raw wheat germ, beans—especially soybeans—sunflower seeds, peanuts, fresh peanut butter, and brown rice.

Also important for hair health and beauty are:

Sulphur, an essential mineral for strong, thick, vibrant hair. Abundant in most high-protein foods, organic sulphur is also found in cauliflower, turnips, cabbage, Brussels sprouts, onions, and garlic. Be careful, though, not to overcook sulphur foods. The less cooking, the more sulphur.

Vitamin B-complex, the secret of growing hair. It, too, is prevalent in the high-protein foods. And remember that most B-vitamins work as teams: a deficiency in one leads to imbalance in another. Also bear in mind that strong black coffee destroys these vital vitamins.

Vitamin C, which strengthens the capillary walls where nutrition passes to your hair follicles. This vitamin is plentiful in citrus fruits, mangoes, strawberries, bananas, pineapple, cherries, melons, peaches, apples, and most green, leafy vegetables.

Vitamin A, for sheen and anti-dandruff protection. Fish-liver oil is one of the richest sources. So are other livers and dark-green leafy vegetables.

In addition to sulphur, there are other minerals that fortify the hair. Iodine promotes normal growth. So does chlorine, which also removes poisons from the system. Zinc and silicon help to keep hair strong and thick.

That is why, in addition to a well-balanced diet, it is important to include vitamin-mineral supplements to your health and beauty program.

One of the most important substances to include in a lovely, healthy hair regime is golden cold-pressed vegetable oil, such as safflower, soy, or sunflower. Each provides lecithin, a nutrient necessary for every hair-building cell.

Like the rest of your body, hair does not need sugar, white flour, or alcohol. Only a limited amount of carbohydrates is required—the quality carbohydrates obtained from natural whole grains, dry legumes (beans of all sorts), fresh vegetables or fruits, and natural brown rice.

With foods containing all of these nutrients, you can plan nourishing meals for your hair and it will respond with a flourishing fringe.

SCALP STIMULATION: BRINGING OUT HAIR SHINE

Your hair can also benefit from certain "exercises." Foremost among them is brushing, which stimulates your oil-secreting glands. Correct brushing also distributes the oils evenly, deep massages the scalp, and cleans the surface of dirt, dead skin, and dandruff.

The proper way to brush hair is from scalp to ends, in the direction of the hair's fall. But don't overdo it. The old standard "100 strokes daily" can be excessive for hair that is not in peak condition, causing hair loss and tangled or split ends. Thirty or less strokes per day should be your maximum. What counts is regularity, not quantity.

Brush firmly but gently, making sure that the bristles touch the scalp. But don't dig into this sensitive area. The purpose is to stimulate—not irritate.

A brush with rounded tips made of soft, natural bristles is safest and most effective. Able to penetrate even the thickest hair, its bristle tips will not cause damage to dry hair. Nylon bristles should be shunned because of their rough ends.

To maximize the benefit of brushing, use only a clean hairbrush. Wash both your brush and comb at least twice a week in warm, soapy water.

Another exercise to stimulate circulation is a gentle finger massage. Sit down and prop your elbows on a table. Then spread all ten fingers on your scalp and rotate in a slow circular movement for a few seconds. The object is to move only the scalp—not your fingers. Cover the whole scalp—including forehead, temples, above your ears, and at the base of your neck.

Going bareheaded is another simple way to stimulate hair. Your scalp, after all, is skin, and it needs to breathe. Tight wigs and hats not only cause excessive perspiration, they also inhibit circulation. Well-fitting headgear should be worn, however, during extremes of cold and sunlight.

SHAMPOOING: CLEANING YOUR CURLS

Regular shampooing is the only way to keep your hair beautifully clean and to prevent a greasy look. Two to three times a week is average if you live in a large polluted city. If you have excessively oily hair, there is no harm in washing it daily. But avoid too-strong shampoos, which can cause tangling and dryness.

Work in the shampoo all over your head—gently. Make sure you include the hairline all around, since makeup and grease collect there. Use very warm but not hot water for washing, and cool water for rinsing. It takes at least ten minutes to rinse hair thoroughly. You'll know you've removed all the shampoo when your hair "squeaks" with pulling.

To shampoo in hard water, dissolve a teaspoonful of Borax in a gallon of water, and use this for lathering and rinsing. You can also try a commercial water softener or use bottled spring water.

Dry hair will benefit more if pre-treated with olive or castor oil for about 20 minutes prior to shampooing. Saturate the scalp with warm oil and wrap the hair in a hot towel. Then rinse with cold water and wash with a protein-enriched shampoo.

Oily hair should be treated to shampoos that contain alcohol, not additional oils. A protein-based shampoo made especially for oily hair will prove the most beneficial.

Since most shampoos are essentially alkaline, make sure you choose one that also contains acidic pH properties. Excessive alkalinity can make hair dull and unmanageable.

Since hair is basically protein, a protein-enriched lather will coat the hair shaft, giving an illusion of fullness. Remember, though, the best protein "treatment" comes from within. Protein shampoo may make the hair shaft more resistant to breakage, but it doesn't actually impart protein to the hair itself.

Here's a *money-saving shampoo tip*. Most commercial shampoos are heavily concentrated. You can save money and get better results by diluting them—four parts water to one part shampoo. This also combats detergent buildup that dulls hair, as undiluted shampoos are difficult to rinse out.

To find the perfect shampoo for yourself takes experimenting. Buy various samples and try them out before purchasing a larger, more expensive bottle. Many discount houses package their own shampoos, which are far less expensive yet equal in quality to the name brands.

To be certain that the acid nature of your hair is restored, even after washing with a pH-balanced shampoo, it is wise to use an apple cider vinegar rinse. This will eliminate oil and soapy film you might have missed with plain water. Simply mix two tablespoons of the vinegar with one pint of warm water and pour slowly over your head. Top it off with a cool, plain water rinse.

Since this mixture tends to darken light hair, blondes should use only one tablespoon of vinegar with a quart of warm water. Or try a refreshing lemon rinse: the strained juice of one lemon added to a pint of warm water, followed by a cold-water rinse.

These recipes, easy and inexpensive, can replace commercial and cream rinses. They make hair shine by restoring its natural gloss.

If you have problem hair (dullness, split ends, frizzies, snarled or limp hair) conditioners with added proteins—such as balsam, milk, egg white, gelatin, lecithin, and soya—will bind with the hair and give the appearance of body.

Or you can apply one of these simple recipes from your own kitchen:

1. Mix a cup of milk, two beaten egg whites, or unflavored gelatin with your shampoo. Even better, add some liquid protein, available in many health-food stores.

2. Mix real mayonnaise (not salad dressing) with a tablespoon of liquid protein and leave on the hair for up to an hour, depending on how dry it is. Following this treatment, shampoo with a protein-enriched brand and rinse with the apple cider vinegar recipe.

If your hair is extremely brittle and dried out, try this simple concoction:

½ oz. wheat-germ oil
3 oz. liquid protein
½ oz. apple cider vinegar
½ oz. glycerine (available at pharmacies)

Mix well and apply to hair AFTER shampooing. Leave on for a half-hour, then rinse thoroughly. This helps restore the natural chemical balance of your hair.

Is beer a good conditioner? Hardly. Beer is a carbohydrate, which can't give the hair anything except a boozy smell. Forget those old wives' tales that it adds body.

A final warning: it is possible to get *too much* protein build-up, especially from superficial commercial protein conditioners. If you have no hair problem, don't overdo the protein. It can mat your hair, make it sticky, greasy-looking, and hard to comb.

DRYING YOUR HAIR: FLUFFING YOUR REGAL RUFF

The greatest danger in drying is excessive heat. This is especially true if you wash your hair every day and blow-dry it afterwards.

Overuse of any hot-air hair dryer can make your hair brittle and dull. Don't use a blow-dryer which has more than 1,000 watts, and never use one daily.

The same advice applies to hot combs, heated electric

rollers, and curling irons. Those that employ heated and/or conditioning mists are better than dry-setting models because the moisture counteracts the drying effect. For greater safety, spray a protein-based product on the hair before drying it to coat and protect it from the hazards of extreme heat.

CUTTING AND STYLING: SHAPING YOUR TRESSES

Though length and shape are matters of personal taste, it is best to work within your hair's own capabilities. If you try to fight its nature, you will probably end up with damaged, lifeless hair.

A good haircut not only suits your facial structure and life-style—it also allows your hair to do what comes naturally. It is a cut that does not need constant upkeep.

Naturally wavy or curly hair is easiest to maintain when short. Long hair needs to be blunt-cut regularly to trim off split ends. Fly-away hair demands a short, chin-length blunt cut to keep the baby-fine hair in place.

The right cut and style can make your eyes look bigger, your nose less prominent, or balance other less-than-perfect features. The best style for you is not necessarily the one worn by a TV or movie queen. It is the one that works best into your daily routine without taking up an undue amount of your time.

If you use hair spray, keep it far away from your eyes. Excessive spray also attracts grime, requiring more frequent washing followed by a cider vinegar or lemon rinse.

It isn't necessary to spend a lot of money on styling aids. You can make your own wave-setting lotion, for example, using flaxseed obtained from a health-food store. Boil one cup of ground or whole flaxseed in three cups of water, and then dilute to the desired consistency. Strain before using. (Discard seeds or add them to cooked cereal.)

You can also use fresh skim milk as a mild wave-set. For a stronger hold, first apply wheat-germ oil. Then rinse with vinegar solution. This adds a definite bounce for those who want hair with body.

Permanents are another way of adding body to limp hair. But much of their success depends on the texture of your hair. Poor results usually occur with fine, limp, wiry, or brittle hair. Again, the hair's natural instinct prevails.

If you wish to straighten your hair's natural wave or curl, I recommend petrolatum-based pomades. Hot-pressing (combing with a heated metal comb) can be damaging to hair and scalp, while chemical straighteners contain caustic ingredients. If you feel you *must* use a chemical product, stick with the type called "curl relaxers," since they are least damaging to the hair.

COLOR: A LITTLE GOES A LONG WAY

There's nothing like a new, glamorous color change to give hair an added beauty boost. An exciting new shade can accent your hair style, enhance your skin tone, enrich the color of your eyes, and highlight your features.

There are many possibilities. You can go lighter or darker, enrich your own color by highlighting, or cover up graying hair. But you should not strive for every-strand-the-same-color, since natural hair coloring is never so uniform.

"Natural" is the key word for hair color. By using natural vegetable bleaches and organic dyes, you avoid possible cancer-causing elements and allergens coming in contact with your scalp. Herbs for the hair are obtainable in most pharmacies and health-food stores.

For light or graying hair, here are two do-it-yourself, natural hair darkeners:

Sage Tea Darkener

4 tbsp. ordinary tea leaves and grounds
1 tbsp. dried sage leaves

Simmer ingredients in one pint of water for half an hour. Strain, saving only the liquid. Massage into hair four or five times weekly, until gray gradually dis appears.

Herbal Hair Darkener

1 oz. sage leaves
1 oz. rosemary herb

Add one pint of water and simmer for half an hour. Strain. With cotton pad, massage throughout the hair. Start with five weekly applications. As hair begins to darken, reduce the frequency gradually.

The following two recipes are for blonde hair coloring:

Chamomile Highlight Rinse

4 tablespoons dried chamomile flowers
1 pint water

Boil 30 minutes, strain, and cool. Pour over head, catching the remains in a basin. Repeat several times.

Blonde Recharger

1 tablespoon licorice root
2 tablespoons oat straw
Sprinkle of saffron

Just barely cover with water and boil. Then strain and rinse already shampooed hair with the infusion. Allow to remain on hair until next shampoo.

For the woman who wishes reddish highlights, henna, a non-irritating, permanent dye, is available in most stores. You just mix the leaves of this African bush in a bowl with water and apply as a rinse or paste. Allow it to stay on your hair until the desired shade is reached.

Natural organic dyes and rinses present no danger to your health. Their drawbacks are few:

Exact shades cannot be guaranteed. They depend on your own hair pigmentation, its condition, previous treatment, and other variables. And because natural dyes are not as fast acting as chemical colorings, more applications are necessary to achieve the desired results.

Their advantages are obvious:

Because herbal and vegetable dyes work gradually, you never have to fear a too drastic change. And, of course, they are a safe alternative to the harsh, chemical dyes which can lead to damaged, overbleached hair and irritated scalps.

A practical suggestion: Before attempting any new hair coloring (or hair style for that matter), it is advisable to spend a bit of time in a store trying on wigs of various colors and shades to see which is best for you.

Also to keep in mind: Hair color should never be a

drastic change from skin color if you want the natural, most flattering effect.

TROUBLED TRESSES: DAMAGE AND HAIR LOSS

Your hair needs your help to ward off the effects of the elements—especially during summer, when the sun's rays can overdry. Cover your hair if you plan to be out in the sun for an extended length of time, and use a natural conditioning treatment to perk up dry hair. Trimming off unsightly frayed ends will also improve your appearance.

Daily swimming in a chlorinated pool poses special problems. Algicides interact with chlorine to leave a greenish deposit on blonde hair. Since there is no simple home remedy for such discoloration, you must wear a bathing cap to prevent this disaster.

When humidity gives you the frizzies, use a non-sticky protein conditioner to improve manageability. If your hair is long enough to braid, wear it up. But don't make the ponytail too tight; excessive tension could cause premature hair loss.

Falling, thinning hair is a source of major concern for both sexes. It can be caused by certain illnesses and surgery, by excessive use of aspirin, cortisone, anti-coagulation drugs, birth-control pills, amphetamines, diet pills, chemotherapy, or by exposure to radiation. When the cause is removed, the hair usually returns to normal.

Generally, however, hair loss is determined by heredity. While women are rarely threatened by baldness, there's a certain amount of thinning we all undergo as we mature. That's nothing to fear, as long as you give your hair proper treatment, inside and out.

Think of your hair as a friend. When it is in good

health, performing at peak proficiency, it wants to be appreciated and admired, not abused. On occasions when your hair is not up to par, it doesn't want to fight you–it needs only a friendly hand to help regain its potential.

And what potential! With easy, inexpensive care, your hair will give you a lifetime of loyalty–capping your shapely form, framing your soft features ... crowning your beauty.

Chapter XIII

HOW'S YOUR EYE-Q?

Eyes ... windows of the soul—mirrors of the mind.

Eyes ... with a mere glance, they can inspire terror—sadness—love.

Eyes ... their gaze can tell of a woman's innermost needs—her longings—her lusts.

> Drink to me only with thine eyes.
> And I will pledge with mine.

Beautiful eyes have inspired poets, songwriters, and playwrights since time immemorial.

Many years ago, a Russian peasant girl inspired the tearful strains of "Dark Eyes." How many of you remember "Green Eyes"? Or the romantic "Spanish Eyes"? Or "When Irish Eyes Are Smiling"?

That long-ago Russian girl probably never wore a drop of makeup. More than likely, she ate natural foods, yogurt and farm-fresh vegetables. In other words, a healthy girl, whose good health was reflected in her eyes.

Beautiful eyes are a mirror of your total good health. And the right diet is as important to the health of your eyes as it is to the rest of your body.

Vitamin A, often referred to as the "skin vitamin," is also one of the vitamins that help improve your eyesight. So is riboflavin or vitamin B-2. And good eyesight is one of the keys to beautiful eyes.

Liver, kidney, sweetbreads, carrots, yams, apricots, peaches, leafy-green vegetables are some of the foods rich in vitamin A, foods you should eat for soft skin and which will benefit your eyes.

A diet rich in vitamin A strengthens your eyes, helping them adjust quickly to bright light, and easing strain. And this is important because squinting and straining are among the chief causes of wrinkles around your eyes.

Astigmatism, a vision-distorting eye disorder, can contribute to wrinkles and lines because it, too, causes squinting and straining. Research has demonstrated that a diet low in protein may contribute to astigmatism.

Salt-water fish and all varieties of liver are abundant sources of the special kind of protein required by the eyes. Not as valuable, but useful, are milk, natural cheeses, eggs, and nuts.

Do you wear corrective lenses? As my longtime readers know, I believe that too many people depend on eyeglasses as a crutch. Nevertheless, there are some who have no choice.

But in order to look beautiful, some women will frequently go without their glasses—especially when they wish to be more appealing to men. To them I say:

Stop kidding yourself! You may think you can manage, but you'll be squinting and straining, maybe adding damage to your vision, and certainly building lines and wrinkles. Besides, with today's choice of high-fashion frames, the right pair of eyeglasses might even add to your glamour.

What about makeup? Here, also, I have mixed feelings. To me, there is nothing more lovely than a pair of healthy eyes scintillating with their natural radiance and hue. True, some grooming of the brows and lashes can enhance the total aura of those eyes, while shadow and coloring, judiciously applied, might highlight their dominant features.

What I strongly discourage is the use of tins of chemical compounds to hide defects. Vision is a precious possession, and any product applied to your eyelids or to the delicate skin around your eyes should be as pure and natural as possible. Truly sensible eye care, like skin care, begins with products in your kitchen and the pantry shelves.

If you are bothered by a puffy, baggy look in the under-eye area, try chamomile tea instead of foundation and cover-up cream. Chamomile has an astringent quality. It works to heal, not conceal.

Brew the tea strong, and be sure to let it cool a bit. Then saturate cotton pads with the brew and relax for about ten minutes with the pads over your eyes. This treatment will not only tighten the skin around the eyes and reduce the swelling; it's also soothing to tired eyes irritated by big-city smog. If you are the tea-bag type, use the warm bag itself instead of cotton pads.

Chamomile tea is also a refreshing and effective toner for delicate skin tissue. A good idea is to prepare a jarful and keep it handy in the refrigerator. Use it cold and pat it gently on the area around the eyes at least twice a day.

Milk, too, makes an excellent eye soother. Combine

milk and very warm water is equal amounts. Soak a soft cloth or absorbent cotton balls and use as a compress.

For those tiny lines caused by squinting and straining, try a strong tea made of an herb called, coincidentally, eyebright. You can buy it in most health-food stores. Apply the tea with saturated cotton or gauze, for fifteen to twenty minutes.

Another treatment for wrinkles and crepey eyes is vitamin E. Puncture a 200-unit capsule and apply in the morning and at bedtime. In a month's time, you may see some startling results.

For dark circles under the eyes, many women find that a damp compress of grated raw potatoes works wonders. Fold in cheesecloth and leave it in place for about fifteen minutes. Be sure the potatoes are freshly grated. Exposed to air too long, grated potatoes seem to lose their astringent quality.

Or cut open a dried fig and place the insides of the halves under each eye. Figs contain a protein-tenderizing substance that reduces puffiness and dark circles. It sometimes alleviates wrinkles, too.

Puffiness or dark shadows are often caused by eyestrain. Intensive reading and poor lighting are common causes. So is untreated weak vision. Such strain is often relieved by one of these eye-relaxing exercises:

1. Cup your hands over your eyes, creating total darkness. Do not close the eye. Visualize any image that is pleasant to you. Gaze at the image until it starts to fade. Do not strain to hold the image. As it vanishes, close your eyes and relax for about fifteen seconds. Repeat as often as you wish.

2. Focus on an object in your room, twelve to fifteen inches away. Suddenly shift your eyes out the window, focusing on a distant object like a chimney or tower.

Focus back and forth from distant object to room object, five to ten times.

3. Open the eyes wide. Roll them in a large circle, ten seconds to the left, ten to the right. Then close and rest the eyes. No limit on the number of repetitions.

When women on limited beauty budgets are forced to economize on cosmetics, they seem willing to forego all eye products except one: lash lengthener. If you are that hooked on lengtheners, be wary of mascaras claiming to make eyelashes appear longer. There is a danger that some of it will flake off and end up in the eyes, causing a great deal of irritation.

Mascara, in fact, has been the cause of more eye infections and allergies than any other cosmetic. It is unnecessary to load your lashes with mascara to make them appear longer. You can achieve the same results naturally, with *castor oil.* That's right, a few drops of castor oil rubbed gently into your lashes nightly, then removed with tissue. Don't wash it off; it's best to leave a little working through the night. Castor oil darkens the tips to create the longer appearance, and you won't need tons of it, as you do mascara. For greater sheen, steep a washed lemon peel in an ounce of castor oil for three days. Then apply.

However, if you insist on using wasteful mascaras, be careful. Mascara can become contaminated if exposed too long. Some water-based mascaras which don't contain adequate preservatives are breeding grounds for bacteria just a day or so after opening.

False eyelashes can be equally dangerous. If one stray drop of applicating glue gets into the eye, it can cause painful irritation, itching, and eyelids swollen like balloons.

To be really safe, eye cosmetics should never be kept longer than six months; water-based mascaras four months. To retard deterioration, store all cosmetics in a cool place.

Any brush or applicator you use near your eyes should be completely clean, so should your hands. One of the most important beauty rules is: keep your hands away from your eyes. Hands are seldom free of some dirt. Never apply makeup without first washing your hands.

One of the most common habits can be one of the most damaging: moistening cake mascara with saliva. It risks the growth of mouth bacteria on the mascara. Continued application of this contaminated mascara can lead to eye infection. Fortunately, the use of cake mascara has practically vanished into limbo—and a good thing, too.

The same holds true for borrowing another woman's mascara or brush. There is always the chance of inheriting bacteria.

If you use any commercial eye makeup, the so-called hypoallergenic cosmetics are safer than most. Formulated for extra-sensitive skin, they do not contain ingredients known to cause allergic reactions on most women.

When it comes to applying makeup, teenagers can get away with almost anything outlandish. But a woman should be subtle with her cosmetics. She should look like a woman. Her eye makeup should make her eyes the focal point of her other qualities.

There is a vast range of eyeshadow colors in both powder and cream form. Whatever the shade you choose, get it in cream form preferably. The eye area has few oil ducts or sweat glands and is the driest part of your face. Powder tends to cake, making your lids appear crepey. When it does cake, there is always the chance of it getting into your eyes and causing trouble.

Applying eyeliner can also be a tricky business. The right way is to start the line in the center of the lid and work to the outer lash. Then from the inside corner, join the line at the center.

Be careful not to stretch the skin at the outer corner of your eye, because if the skin is not smooth and flat you may end up with a wavy line. When this happens, the liner may cake in that spot and dry the skin even more.

When applying mascara, be sure to brush it on from the base of the lashes right out and over the tips. It's important to brush in the natural direction, the direction in which they grow. Brushing the lashes back and forth can damage the roots.

For the bottom lashes, use the tip of the brush and hold it at an angle. As a finishing touch, apply a bit more mascara to the outside lashes. A woman with naturally blonde lashes can intensify them by using brown or dark blue mascara, and finishing the tips with black.

If you want to give close-set eyes a far-apart look, use a light shade and a darker shade of the same color shadow. Apply the light shade to the first third of the eyelid and the darker shade to the remaining area. The darker shade should be brought a little beyond the outside corner, then blend both shades toward the brow.

If your problem is small, deep-set eyes, you can give them more definition in almost the same way. Use two shades of an eyeshadow, but in this case divide them equally—the lighter shade on the inside, the darker on the outside. Again, bring the dark tone a little beyond the outside corner of the eye.

To be subtle, the shade of eyeshadow you use must complement the color of your eyes and your skintone.

And beware of sun on your eyelids. Skin tissue here is much thinner than on the rest of your face and needs a great deal of protection from the sun.

There is no safe sunscreen for eyelid use, so the best way to handle it is to keep your sunglasses on, even if you do end up with white circles around your eyes. Another method is to cover your eyelids with wet pieces of cotton. This may also leave you with white circles, but subtly applied makeup can correct them.

Take care with any sunscreen product you use on your face. Believe the manufacturer's label when it states: "not to be used near the eyes."

Healthy, subtly made-up eyes can be one of your most important features. They should be, because research estimates that approximately 60 percent of human communication is through gestures and the eyes.

Eyes are indeed "the windows of the soul," because with them you can transmit the most basic and most subtle nuances. An attractive smile does not always represent how you really feel, but the eyes rarely fool anyone.

The pupils of your eyes, for instance, can inform a man whether you are attracted to him. If your reaction is positive, your pupils will dilate and stay that way for quite a while.

More important, your eyes reflect much about your personality. "Drab" ... "lively" ... "bored" ... "inviting" ... these and countless other adjectives are used to describe eyes, the first clue to the total you. They also reveal the state of your health.

And because eyes don't lie, they can't look healthy without the cooperation of a healthy body. By observing the rules for healthful living, you can have your eyes saying: "I am beautiful."

Chapter XIV

DO YOUR HANDS BETRAY YOU?

What can't we do with our hands!

Hands are used to build mighty structures or mold tiny miniatures. They paint portraits—write novels—perform concertos. Every day, hands are engaged in thousands of tasks, large and small, which we take for granted.

But hands also have a subtler function—as your messengers. Each time you reach for an object, shake another person's hand, point out a direction, your hands invite attention to yourself. By merely holding a man's hand, stroking his hair, caressing his face, your hands convey messages of affection, love, longing.

And when your hands are beautiful, they tell the world that you are beautiful all over.

Considering all the work your hands must perform—and the frequent abuse they undergo—is it possible to preserve their natural loveliness? Unquestionably.

No matter what your age or what kind of job you

perform—homemaker, factory or office worker—you don't have to settle for rough, raw-looking hands. There's no reason to let them disintegrate into worn-out, wrinkled flesh masses, covered with telltale age spots.

You can help your hands on a daily basis simply by washing them properly. Which means: don't just stick them under the faucet.

Fill a basin with lukewarm water (if you have hard water, add a softener) and slosh your soap to make a few suds. (Avoid deodorant soap, which contains drying chemicals.) Lather your hands and rub with a nubbly washcloth. Use a cotton-tipped stick under the fingernails. After washing for a full minute, rinse in lukewarm water and dry them thoroughly, pushing back the cuticles each time. Make sure your hands are *really* dry, as dampness can lead to rough, red skin.

For stains or discoloration, apply a little lemon juice after drying. It works gradually to fade most spots that are caused externally.

If your hands are caked with dirt that ordinary soap can't remove, don't automatically reach for a harsh, abrasive cleansing solvent. First try an oatmeal rub. Simply wet your hands and rub them with dry oatmeal, which should whisk away the heavy particles and grime. Then follow the procedure for cleansing the skin and nails.

Cleansing by itself, however, is not sufficient to keep average hands soft and lovely. Hands need additional help because they are constantly exposed to the natural elements, touching dirty objects, reaching into unclean places. And since they have fewer oil cells than your face, they tend to dryness more easily.

Beautiful hands must be guarded against their enemies. Heed the following hints and you will watch your hands grow softer, more smooth:

1. To fight dryness, use moisturizing lotion or

emollient cream every time you put your hands in water—after doing dishes, swimming, even after baths and showers. A small bottle or jar of moisturizer should be stationed next to every sink and basin in your home and carried in your purse to work.

2. For protection against caustic chemicals, wear rubber gloves when using scouring pads, power cleaners, and harsh ammonia. Wear them, if possible, while doing dishes—otherwise, use a dish brush to spare your hands the ordeal of long immersion in dishwater. It's a good idea, in fact, to don gloves for all kitchen work.

3. To prevent the ravages of inclement and cold weather, always wear gloves outdoors. Put them on *before* you leave the house—*before* they start to dry and chap.

If chapping has already begun, your hands can be helped by equal parts of glycerine and rose-water, or with vitamin E cream or lotion. Keep them out of water as much as possible. At bedtime, apply pure lanolin or petroleum jelly and wear clean white, cotton gloves to bed.

For ordinary redness, develop the habit of keeping your forearm up, with your hands held high so the blood will drain down. If you practice this whenever you sit down to relax—while watching TV, for example—the redness will lessen. The treatment for chapped hands will also help, as will liquid protein, cocoa butter, plain butter, or margarine—applied at night so it can work to improve the skin surface while you sleep.

Other home remedies for redness include soaking your hands in a mixture of honey and unsweetened orange juice for five minutes, nightly massaging with lanolin and almond oil. Either procedure seals in natural moisture, making the hands softer and more alluring.

For cold, clammy hands, try daily gentle massages to improve blood circulation. Starting at the elbow, knead and press lightly down your forearm, working over your hands and fingers until there is a slight tingle.

Here are some simple movements to develop supple and relaxed hands:

First, vigorously shake your hands, loosely from the wrists, to the count of 25. Next, pretend you are playing the piano, wiggling all your fingers up and down in the air for a minute or two.

Then clench your fingers into a tight fist for another count of 25, followed by holding the fingers out, fan-shaped, for a count of 30.

Finally, leaving one hand in position, tug at the fingers in an outward direction, then massage inward, as if trying on gloves. Do this with each hand.

These exercises, in combination with proper nutrition, will stimulate a warm, rosy glow. Your hands will become softer, more graceful—more kissable.

NAIL BEAUTY

Long, strong fingernails are more than a mere beauty feature. These "horny" extensions of the skin are actually barometers of your total health—a measure of the beauty from within. Doctors can often tell the condition of your general health by observing your fingernails.

Like hair, nails are mostly protein (keratin) with a touch of of calcium, phosphorus, and trace minerals. So a wholesome diet—high in protein, low in carbohydrates—is essential to fortify weak, splitting fingernails.

When it comes to their fingernails, most women are guilty of overcare. You may be doing more harm than good if you constantly change nail polish, colors, push back cuticles too often, or overbuff.

Nail polish remover is acetone based and therefore

extracts oil or fat from the nails. By using it daily to remove old nail enamel, you subject your fingernails to a slow-but-sure drying process which will ultimately leave them very brittle.

The best tender and loving care you can lavish on your nails is a five-minute soak in half a cup of wheat-germ oil, as part of your weekly manicure. On a daily basis, you can rub either wheat-germ oil or vitamin E on the nails for a minute or two, then rinse with warm water.

Daily prodding the cuticle with hand objects—even the standard orangewood stick—disturbs the very base of the nail, the only living part, which is susceptible to infection. Pushing the cuticle back too hard often results in white spots—bruises caused by air sneaking in between the nail layers, where it doesn't belong.

If you insist on using an orangewood stick, then wrap a bit of cotton ball around the tip. A damp towel, however, will do the job just as well—especially right after a bath or shower when the cuticle is softest.

To prevent red, inflamed areas around your fingers, be careful when wielding knives or cuticle scissors. Trim only hangnails and jagged tears in the cuticle—don't hack around the edge of the cuticle itself. Use a cuticle remover to loosen any adhering bits.

For maintaining long, sturdy, pretty fingernails, it would benefit you to develop these habits:

1. Use wheat-germ oil, vegetable oil or vitamin E oil to rub the cuticle every day. This will prevent brittleness and drying.

2. Learn to pick up objects with your whole hand, not with the tips of your fingers.

3. Never pry up thumbtacks or jewelry clips or open containers with your fingernails. Use the edge of a knife. Undo knots with a pin, pencil, or other appropriate tool.

4. Dial the telephone with your knuckles, a plastic dialer, or the eraser end of a pencil. Avoid jarring the fingernail when flicking light switches.

5. If you don't have gloves and must perform a dirty job—like potting plants—sink your nails into a bar of soap to embed some under each nail. This will trap grimy, black build-up, which later can be dissolved away under water.

6. Wear nail polish on days when you clean house, type, or perform any other task that adds stress to your fingernails. Polish protects the nails from snagging and breaking.

Most women can't afford the time or cost of a professional weekly manicure, but everyone can learn how to do the same basic steps. With a bit of practice, you can achieve beautiful results right in the comfort of your own home.

Set aside a leisurely hour once a week, perhaps while watching TV. Assemble the following kit:

oily nail polish remover
cotton cleansing pads
cuticle remover
cuticle scissors
emery boards
coffee filter paper and nail cement
  (or commercial nail-repair kit)
nail polish (liquid or paste),
  color of your choice
base coat
sealer
buffer

To make life easier for yourself, these items should be stored in a single container for convenient weekly access. You will also need:

wheat-germ oil
emollient cream
hydrogen peroxide (if dark under nail tip)
lemon juice
white iodine

You are now ready for your nail-beautifying treatment:

1. Heat a half cup of wheat-germ oil in a saucepan.
2. While waiting, remove old nail polish, using cotton pad saturated with polish remover.
3. Wash with mild soap and dry. Apply emollient hand lotion.
4. Push back cuticles with a warm damp washcloth or cotton-tipped stick.
5. File each nail at a 45° angle with emery board, in an upward direction only. (Sawing back and forth against the grain weakens the nail. So does filing too close on the sides.) Stick to shaping a tapered tip that extends above the finger. Make sure there are no rough edges.
6. Wipe each nail with a damp cotton pad to remove any fine dust.
7. Retrieve the warmed oil and place in a small, deep bowl on your lap. Immerse fingernails in the oil for a five-minute soak. (This is where TV comes in handy, to while away the time.)
8. After the five minutes, remove your hands and wipe off excess oil with a cotton pad. Apply lemon juice to each nail to restore the acid mantle.
9. Now it's time to apply an oily cuticle remover. Follow the package directions.
10. With cuticle scissors, trim hangnails and loose cuticles and apply white iodine over the nail and surrounding flesh.

11. Apply emollient cream to hands and nails.

12. Clean under nails with a bit of cotton on a stick, and apply hydrogen peroxide.

13. Wash your hands thoroughly and dry them.

14. If you intend to use nail polish afterward, patch any tear in the nail, using a commercial nail-repair kit. Or cut and shape your own patch out of coffee filter paper and affix with nail cement. This could save a nail that might otherwise have torn off.

15. Now you are ready for polish. You can apply paste-polish and buff in one direction, for the natural look, or follow these steps for properly applied nail color:

16. Apply base coat of clear, oil-based polish underneath the nail and over the edge. Cover the top with two coats, allowing two minutes between coats.

17. To polish with enamel, start in the middle of the nail and coat down to the base, avoiding the cuticle, then back up to the tip. Apply in slow strokes, using only a little bit on the brush, and allow two minutes of drying time between first and second coats. Avoid "frosted" enamel polish, which is drying to fingernails.

18. Add a clear sealer for protection against chipping. *Avoid nail hardeners that contain formaldehyde.* This harsh chemical can cause discoloration, bleeding under the nails, and loss of the nail itself.

19. With a buffer, shine your nails up to a beautiful sparkle. Don't buff too hard or you will burn the nail. Buff only in one direction.

Let the color of your nails express your individual style. You can go light and natural, match color to your wardrobe, add designs and decals, or duplicate your lipstick color.

The standard for beautiful fingernails is ten even nails, with tips extending one third the length of the pink part. Avoid overly long, catlike claws; a sensible length is easier to maintain than exaggerated talons.

Together, beautifully soft hands and homegrown, lovely fingernails add up to a statement about *you*. Their glorious condition conveys to the world that you care about them—about yourself—about others.

No matter what your age, you can take steps to preserve your hands and nails from the ravages of time. With proper diet and external care you can recapture, maintain, and enhance their natural allure.

And that's the way it should be: lovely hands that reach out to convey a message . . . the message that you are beautiful all over.

Chapter XV

FOR FEET'S SAKE–PUT YOUR BEST FOOT FORWARD

Would you believe there's a better than 50–50 chance that those deepening wrinkles around your temples, those crevices and furrows between your eyes, and the tightened lines around your mouth are caused by your feet? Impossible? No, not really.

To most people, it comes as a surprise that their feet are their number-one "wrinkle maker." That's because nerve endings in abused or overtired feet send pain signals as fast as a telegraph system–right up to cloud your countenance with a frown. And hurting feet register in your posture too.

Sore, aching feet can cause you to hunch your shoulders to obtain relief. With chronic foot trouble you are inclined to bend your knees to ease the pressure. This can lead to curving of the spine to accommodate the displaced weight.

And you thought your feet didn't need special attention!

All these years you've been cramming them into fashionable high-heel shoes. And at what price? Constant wearing of high-heel shoes (three inches or over) takes a slow toll on your health and appearance. It is the source of many a backache, swollen legs, and sore feet. And the situation becomes progressively worse when you remove the offending shoes, because you force the now-contracted leg muscle to stretch much further than it's accustomed. So even walking barefoot or in low-heel shoes becomes painful.

Excessive wearing of high heels can also lead to lordosis, an exaggerated forward curvature of the spine.

If you never before realized that your feet could create so much havoc in your pro-beauty program, quite likely you also didn't know that there *is* a proper treatment plan for your feet. They too can be beautiful!

You may think that no one ever notices your feet, since they are generally covered. Yet you go barefoot in summer in the yard. Or at the beach, You show parts of your foot whenever you wear sandals. And you often take off your shoes at home or at the office to relax.

An unkempt-looking foot is a real turn-off. Rough, red heels, calloused toes, and sweaty, odorous feet don't belong on a beauty-conscious woman. They do distract from an otherwise gorgeous appearance.

So stop dragging your feet. Start now to follow these guidelines for healthier, prettier feet:

1. Never wear the same shoes two days in a row—allow time for the moisture in the shoes to evaporate.
2. Give your feet an air bath: go barefoot for an hour at a time. This stimulates circulation.
3. Change your pantyhose or socks every day.
4. Avoid excessively tight-topped knee-high socks,

which impede blood flow to the feet.

5. Apply vegetable oil to the toenails every night. The natural oil penetrates the nail (which is protein) and prevents cracking and splitting.
6. Practice the proper way to clean your fabulous feet:
   a) Scrub foot top and bottom with soap, using hand brush with moderately stiff bristles.
   b) Use a soft tissue to clean between toes.
   c) Rinse, and while wet, rub heel and ball of foot with pumice stone, using a rotary motion. This reduces rough spots.
   d) Vigorously dry feet (a form of massage to stimulate circulation).
   e) Dry well between toes—sprinkle foot powder.
   f) Push back cuticles while they're soft.
   g) Rub in moisturizing cream.
   h) Dust with talcum powder.
7. Check your shoes for repairs. Run-down heels and worn-out soles can lead to foot troubles.
8. Pamper your precious feet with a weekly pedicure. Observe as many of the following suggestions as possible:
   a) Remove toenail polish.
   b) Follow procedure for the foot bath, omitting the final talc.
   c) Clean under the toenails with an orangewood stick wrapped in cotton.
   d) Apply vegetable oil to toenails.
   e) Apply cream and massage for 10 minutes. Consider using a skin cream rich in vitamin E. Or pierce a 400-unit vitamin E capsule and squeeze a drop on each toenail, rubbing in well. Use regularly and notice how the surrounding skin will improve.

f) Remove excess cream and oil with cleansing tissues.
g) Cut and file toenails square. Don't try to round the corners, as you would for fingernails.
h) Remove dead cuticle with commercial cuticle remover. For ragged cuticles, apply vitamin-E oil, which promotes quick healing.
i) Wash off any excess and dry foot.
j) Place cotton balls between toes and adorn each toenail with two lustrous coats of polish.

9. Never use a razor on any foot disorder (corn or callous). It could lead to infection.
10. Learn to encase your foot in comfort: select well-fitting shoes.
    a) The shoe should extend one-half inch longer than your big toe.
    b) The shoe should be roomy at the broadest part of the foot.
    c) The shoe should fit snugly at the heel, under the arch, and over the instep.
    d) Try on both shoes! Each foot is a slightly different size.
    e) Always make sure the shoes you intend to purchase—especially tennis shoes—have arches. Flat sneakers do damage to your foot's natural arch and tire your feet rapidly.
    f) Never . . . repeat, NEVER . . . buy shoes that are too tight with the thought that they will expand with use.

To help beautify your feet, you have to be able to identify and eliminate foot problems. If you catch them in the bud, you will not only save yourself the cost of a visit to the chiropodist, but many added wrinkles and many hours of foot-wrenching pain.

Corns are caused by ill-fitting shoes. If a shoe fits too tight, it presses the feet; if too loose, it causes friction. The best treatment is prevention, but if you spot a hardened area building up, try this home remedy:

For three consecutive nights, soak the area in warm water for 15 minutes. Next, apply liquid corn remover or salve only to the corn itself. Or use a cotton ball soaked with witch hazel. Wear a corn plaster between soakings. After the third treatment, you should be able to lift out the core of the corn. If not, time to see the chiropodist or podiatrist.

Callouses are another foot-beauty blight. These scaly, thick skin masses can really detract from a graceful foot shape. They are generally caused by poor-fitting shoes, faulty posture, weak arches, or foot strain. To eradicate them at their early stage, use pumice stone to remove the top layer and try the treatment recommended for corns to soften the deeper layers.

Ingrown toenails are caused by shoes that cramp the toes, or by cutting the toenail outer edges too short.

This painful condition can be prevented by cutting toenails straight across or slightly crescent-shaped, leaving the outer edges longer than the middle.

If you are plagued by a painful, unsightly bunion, no home remedy is available. Use of adhesive padding, well-fitting shoes, and witch hazel compresses can provide some relief, but surgery on the joint is the usual way to correct the big-toe bone displacement.

Blisters are a rather common foot problem caused by chafing and pressure on the skin. It is best to leave a blister alone, since the unbroken skin is its best protection from infection. If it breaks, the loose skin should be trimmed off with sterilized manicure scissors.

Swollen feet are uncomfortable as well as unbecoming. Prevention is obviously the best cure. If you know you will be doing a lot of walking, be sure to wear comfortable shoes. Bloated ankles and puffy, discolored feet detract from the loveliness of any woman.

If your feet do swell for any reason, don't ignore this distress signal. Prop them higher than hip level and wrap them in a wet towel for five minutes a day. If the swelling persists, consult your doctor.

For tired, aching feet that long to be soothed, try immersing them for a 3-minute soak. Use warm water and a handful of Epsom salts or baking soda. Another variation uses witch hazel with a few added ice cubes.

Rinse your feet with cool water, then dry and massage in moisturizing cream for ten minutes. If you can prop your feet up for another ten minutes, all the better. Your feet will love you for it.

To relax your friendly feet (with the added bonus of stimulating circulation) try a quick and easy bottle exercise. Simply press your bare foot down on a large round bottle and roll it back and forth. Give each foot about two minutes. This simple exercise lovingly massages the muscles which run the length of the foot.

The same procedure, using a tennis ball instead, makes a wonderful massage for the muscles across the ball of the foot. Practiced daily, this easy method can work wonders with overworked feet.

Using a vibrator on the lower instep and ankles will also relax tense foot muscles after a hard day on your feet.

Sometimes, unknowingly, you put your foot into more than it can handle. By this I mean putting your *bare* feet into chemical-laden leather shoes, or into plastic shoes that cause your feet to sweat excessively. Always wear some sort of stockings to prevent shoe irritation.

If you're good to your feet, they will be good to you and serve you well.

Next to your heart, your feet carry the greatest load of any part of your body. Statisticians figure you will walk 65,000 miles in a lifetime—enough to travel around the world 2½ times!

That's reason enough to take good care of them. They make a vital contribution to your appearance—and can make or break those unnecessary facial wrinkles that detract from a beautiful face.

Break loose from any old nasty habits of abusing your hard-working born-to-be-beautiful feet! (Have you ever seen a baby with rough, scaly feet?)

You can be footloose and fancy-free whether you are shopping, dancing, or hiking through the Alps—if only you take good care of your feet.

You can walk gracefully and erect, knowing you can keep your feet both healthy and beautiful.

Chapter XVI

WHICH FRAGRANCE IS YOU?

Glamorous.
Mysterious.
Exciting.
Sensuous.
Exotic.

Words with the power to evoke images. Words that have become almost synonymous with beauty. Small wonder these words are used to describe the effect of perfume and cologne on the senses.

Such is the power of words and the human sense of smell, it almost becomes a puzzle: did the word evoke the scent or the scent evoke the word?

Say that something is *mysterious*, and to someone's mind will come a scene of the Far East and the scent of sandalwood.

Exotic often conjures up a South Seas island and a beautiful wahine with flowers in her hair. To some, the word *sensuous* brings a glimpse of satin sheets and a whiff of a warm, heady aroma.

And it works conversely. The hint of a certain scent will often remind us of another time, another place, an exciting occasion, a never-to-be-forgotten summer evening, or that very special person.

Women have been making themselves more feminine, glamorous, and unforgettable with perfume for centuries. The Romans, who practically invented bathing and the art of sensuous living, also invented liquid and solid perfumes and ointments, which combined as many as twenty different ingredients. They used these perfumes and ointments generously in their baths and rubbed them into their skins.

When the Roman legions marched through Europe, they built public baths everywhere. But when the Romans were defeated, their baths were destroyed. And the victorious populace became a stinking lot!

No wonder the use of perfume became essential. Today's consumer, who adds perfume or cologne as the finishing touch after bath or shower, may find it shocking to learn that for a very long time Europeans used perfume to cover up for baths they never took.

Reservoirs to hold our water supplies, the advent of indoor plumbing, the ease of that daily bath or shower give us the opportunity to use perfume as it was really meant to be used. Like the Romans, we can take full advantage of the "magic" a good scent carries, using it to enhance and not to hide something. Perfume gives us the luxury of feeling fresh, alive, warm, exciting, ultra-feminine.

Oh, yes—and masculine too! Fragrances for men and women, except obviously heavy floral scents, are almost interchangeable. I know of one woman who found her husband's new cologne preferable to what she had been using and now buys a bottle for each of them. Instead of clashing, their fragrances complement each other.

Yes, complement—for nothing can spoil a mood between you and your man more than incompatible fragrances. It's difficult to get close to someone with whom you don't blend.

Most fragrances fall into one of the several basic types, according to their chemical compositions:

ORIENTAL fragrances use musk, civet, and ambergris as fixatives to produce a sultry, exotic, often heady aroma.

SPICY fragrances combine pungent ingredients like cinnamon, clove, ginger, vanilla, and spicy flowers such as carnation.

FRUITY blends usually have a citrus base and a hint of the refreshing scent of orange, lemon, apricot, peach, sometimes tangerine, and a touch of grapefruit.

FLORAL BOUQUETS are an intricate blend of a variety of flowers, with no one scent predominating.

SINGLE FLORALS have the dominant note of one flower, such as rose, gardenia, jasmine, or lily of the valley.

WOODSY-MOSSY fragrances are a mixture of rosewood, sandalwood, cedarwood, and balsam, combined with ferns and herbs. The resulting scent is reminiscent of the fresh, outdoorsy aroma of a forest.

Of course, it's one thing to know about basic ingredients and quite another to figure out which is most appropriate for you. Of the many and varied fragrances offered by department stores and boutiques, how do you decide which one is "just right"?

When you go to shop for perfume or cologne *do it alone*. Finding the right fragrance is a very personal experience. It must please you and you alone. You don't want to be influenced by another person's preferences. If you are with someone who is becoming bored or is in a rush, you may easily make the wrong choice.

Selecting a perfume should be done slowly and calmly. Sniffing directly from the bottle won't give you the true character of the scent. Nor will trying out a few testers haphazardly.

The proper way to sample fragrance is to put a drop or two on the wrist at the pulse point. Don't use your fingers, ask the salesperson to apply them for you. One sample on each wrist and possibly one more scent at the crook of one elbow. It's not wise to sample more than three at one time, because your nose may get mixed up and the fragrances will all smell alike.

Once they've been applied, give them ample opportunity to interact with your skin oils. At this point, it's a good idea to go browsing in another part of the store for about ten or fifteen minutes. When you return to the perfume counter, you should be able to evaluate the different scents and make the right decision.

You'll know when you've found the right fragrance, because something wonderful happens. Your metabolism, your body chemistry, combine with the perfume or cologne to produce that particularly delightful aroma that makes you feel feminine, confident, and glamorous. The scent that adds to your total beauty. The aroma that is you.

If you do your fragrance shopping in the summertime, the right decision will include your choice in cologne form also. Perfume, the most concentrated fragrance, is greatly affected by warm, sultry weather. The higher the temperature, the more potent it will smell. If your choice is one of the heavier scents, it can become overpowering as the temperature rises. That's because the skin surface becomes more oily as the heat stimulates the sebaceous glands. Oily skin holds fragrance longer.

Cologne, less expensive and far lighter than perfume, is ideal for hot-weather use. It is actually the best choice for year-round, because it never seems too heavy. Use it in all the strategic places: behind your ears, on your wrists, between your breasts. Then splash it lavishly on your arms, legs, shoulders, and belly; let the warmth of your body do the rest.

Once you have found your special fragrance, it's a good idea to collect it in its many forms. Whether you are using bath powder to soothe and refresh your skin, or an after-bath moisturizer, it should be in your fragrance, if possible. While soaps, bath products, and colognes have a much lower intensity of fragrance, together they have a great impact on the senses.

It is a mistake to layer yourself with a near gagging variety of fragrances. As one male friend of mine put it, "Nothing turns me off faster than a woman who smells like a walking cosmetics counter!" Starting with your bath, your aim should be to have everything harmonize, to surround yourself with a single fragrance aura.

Bathing has once again become the time for relaxing and beautifying that it was in Roman times. While luxuriating in the bath, you can soothe and glamorize yourself with many products scented to suit you and your man. Give perfume a chance to work its magic, and it can lead to a more exciting evening than you ever planned.

Following are some of the products to turn a bath into something more than mere bathing:

BATH OIL in liquid, spray, or capsule form soothes and perfumes the skin.

BATH BEADS AND CRYSTALS add a light perfume to the water and act as water softeners.

BATH AND SHOWER GELS add a delicate fragrance to the skin, while acting as skin softeners.

BUBBLE BATH—no matter what your age. Relaxing in a tub full of fragrant bubbles is still a lovely way to start or end the day.

AFTER-BATH FRESHENERS are lighter than cologne. Splashed on, the alcohol cools and lightly tones the skin.

AFTER-BATH LOTIONS scent and soothe rough, chapped skin.

If by some chance you've run out of any of these and are preparing for a special evening, a capful or two of cologne in the bathwater will start you off delightfully.

The fragrance aura you have created for yourself can follow and surround you in many interesting and exciting ways. Everything you wear and touch can leave behind a lingering scent that will keep you in someone's mind.

If you spray cologne on padded clothes hangers, your clothes and everything in the closet will soon pick up a touch of the scent.

If you feel your perfume doesn't last long enough, a few drops on a bit of cotton, tucked into your bra, will ensure many hours of warm fragrance.

Cotton shirts will smell delightfully of you if you sprinkle cologne on the ironing board before ironing them.

Do the same before ironing cotton hankerchiefs and your handbag will spill out the aroma every time you open it. It you don't use handkerchiefs, a bit of cologne on a cotton ball, hidden in your handbag, will do the trick.

To keep your special warm scent around you, try rinsing your intimate apparel in water sprinkled with your cologne.

If you've prepared an intimate dinner for two, don't spoil the effect by burning scented candles which may conflict with your fragrance. Instead, put a few drops of your perfume in the melted wax of an ordinary candle and let the heat send the perfume through the room.

A drop of perfumed bath oil on the electric light

bulbs will have the same effect. Or pour a small puddle of cologne into a glass ashtray and light it. When the alcohol has burned off, the air will be redolent with the wafting scent.

And to insure both of you pleasant, fragrant dreams, spray your sheets and pillowcases with cologne whenever you think it is necessary.

Even empty perfume bottles are valuable as long as some scent remains. Don't throw them away; just remove the stopper and tuck a bottle in among your lingerie or in your sweater drawer. Or put them in the linen closet among the towels.

Perfume should be used, not hoarded. It is an expensive waste of money to keep it unused for too long. Use it and enjoy it. Once the bottle has been opened, perfume will start to oxidize and change its character. What smelled delightful in January can look and smell radically different the following August.

Air and light are enemies of perfume, so every time you open the bottle, replace the stopper carefully, even giving it an extra twist. Store it in a relatively cool, dark place.

If you received a gift of a very large bottle of your favorite perfume, the chances of it remaining unaffected by air and light are not very good if you are going to open it every day. It would be best to transfer some of it to a small bottle, using an eye dropper, and reseal the large bottle. Don't forget to put it back in that cool, dark place until it's time for another refill.

MAKING YOUR OWN SCENT

With all the fancy advertising and high prices of perfumes, one gets the impression that its manufacture is an intricate, expensive process. Nothing can be further from the truth. Like the rest of the cosmetics industry, bottled fragrances are grossly overpriced. And while some scents come from unique, faraway sources, others need be no more distant than your local pharmacy.

Home *parfumerie* has other advantages besides the saving of money. Think of the hassle you avoid at department stores, where salespersons are bombarding you from all directions, or at boutiques, where limited selections never leave you quite satisfied. Most important, by experimenting with your own formulas, you can come up with one or more fragrances which are *strictly* you.

The basic ingredients you'll need are alcohol and essential oils. And while I don't advocate vodka for drinking, it does make an excellent alcohol base for your mixtures, because it is odorless.

A fragrant COLOGNE can be made by adding 4 drops oil of lavender, 4 drops oil of rosemary, and 1 drop tincture of ambergris to one-half pint of alcohol and shaking it well. Then mellow the scent; let it age for about two weeks in a dark place.

A delightful PERFUME combines 5 drops tincture of ambergris, 3 drops oil of orange, 4 drops oil of lavender, and 3 drops oil of rosemary with one cup of alcohol. Ambergris adds a hint of warmth and seduction to the scent. Be sure to close the glass container tightly, and since this is perfume, let the mixture age for at least three months.

You may want to try oil of patchouli and oil of rose geranium in your fragrance experiments—but be sure to add 2 to 3 drops of musk to all your blends to help the oils and alcohol mix well and to give the fragrance a "lift."

One of my all-time favorite recipes makes a refreshing unisex SPLASH-ON, perfect for cooling off in summer weather. Its pungent scent evokes memories of tropical breezes and lovely Caribbean damsels. Once again vodka makes the perfect, tingly base.

To 5 ounces of vodka in a glass jar add 1 ounce light rum, ½ teaspoon allspice, ¼ teaspoon orange extract, a few bay leaves, and one stick of cinnamon. Let the mixture stand for about two weeks, but shake it vigorously every now and then. Double or triple the ingredients and you will have enough to use as gifts to both male and female friends.

The above are basic examples. Many, many different oils are available. Try them in varying combinations. Add more of one, less of another. *Experiment!* Your own sense of smell is your best guide as to how much or how little oil or essence to use.

Try them for special occasions or for just-around-the-house wear. Before long, you will have a shelf-full of original fragrances for every need—and suited to your personality.

Where are the best places to apply these perfumes?

Marilyn Margulis, a consultant on natural beauty, recommends that you hit all of these points: behind the knees, the soft skin between the thighs, above the heart, the wrists, the inner arms, the bosom, throat, back of neck, and temples.

Behind the ears? "Absolutely not!" Mrs. Margulis warns. Women do a lot of perspiring in that area, and nothing can kill the desired effect faster than excessive sweat.

Always remember, though: there is no greater "perfume" than the fragrance of fresh, clean, healthy bodies. There is no substitute for soap and water, no scent that can hide the bodily odors caused by faulty nutrition.

Perfume cannot—must not—be a mask or sham. Its true purpose is to enhance and complement the natural smells that label you a woman.

Chapter XVII

HOW TO MAKE ENDS NEAT

(Spot Reducing and Other Exercises)

At last! After months of faithful dieting, you're slimmed down to the 125 pounds you weighed fifteen years ago. You've learned to eat well and control your appetite ... no fear of regaining that excess poundage. You're ready for the big plunge.

You race to the most exclusive shop in your area, try on their most sexy bikini ... and suddenly your whole world falls apart! What happened?

Instead of the svelte body you expected to see in that bikini, you discover you are soft in some places and bulge in others. After you worked so hard on your diet. Could your scale have lied? It's almost as if you haven't shed an ounce!

This is not an uncommon problem, especially among maturing people. Learning to eat well slimmed you down and will keep you slim but because of your life-style you haven't lost weight proportionately. In fact, if it were possible to weigh individual parts of the body, you might find that you actually *gained* a few pounds.

This happens because, untoned after years of disuse, muscles start to atrophy. Muscle fibers shrink and are slowly replaced by fat—in areas which no amount of dieting can improve. Only exercise can reduce the fatty deposits in these spots.

While everyone agrees to the necessity of exercise, most people fight it, convincing themselves that it is boring. They put it off because of the time, the weather, or any number of other excuses. Mostly they feel it's not worth the effort.

Not worth it? Think of some swimmers you know. Do *they* have thick waists or flabby arms, bulging midriffs or flat chests? The great contours you see on swimmers are the end result of consistent exercise that reaches every part of their bodies.

Of course, swimming is not the only way to exercise. It may not be for you. You—and everyone else—need *some* form of exercise to firm you up and tone your muscles. Only then can you say "good-bye" to soft spots. Even those "too thin" areas, like the hollows in your neck and chest, will vanish, giving your body a smooth, curved appearance. But mainly exercise will pare down bumps and bulges that dieting alone couldn't change.

Exercising does not have to be a long drawn-out procedure, and it isn't necessary to over-do. There's no need to work against a deadline. How much you do, or how hard you do it, is not what really counts. The whole point of exercising is to do it regularly. According to Dr. Andrew Myers, an authority on obesity, 10 minutes of mild morning exercise and a 20-minute evening walk could take one pound off you every thirty days—even without a change in eating habits.

A once-or twice-a-week schedule doesn't do much for anyone. Amateur tennis players may have fun, but they're not getting exercise benefits if they don't play often enough. If they don't devote at least three days, spread out over the week, they should exercise in other ways too. The same holds true for all activities.

Let's look now at three basic exercises that give all parts of you a simultaneous workout:

SWIMMING

Swimming is such good exercise because it conditions and relaxes at the same time. It builds what needs building and slims what needs slimming. Which is why you rarely see flat bosoms on women who swim regularly.

You can actually turn your swimming sessions into exercises for specific areas of your body. To trim down a bulgy waistline or bumpy hips and to flatten your tummy, concentrate on the crawl. If your particular problem is flabby arms, perfect your backstoke. As for the breast stroke, it couldn't have a better name. Work on it regularly and you'll soon see what I mean.

If you haven't swam in years, don't suddenly jump in and go for broke. Swimming is strenuous exercise, and some things about you may have changed. Muscles have probably softened and weakened. Your most important muscle, the heart, can be overstrained by an unexpected, unusually strong workout. As with any new exercise, start slowly. It might even be a good idea to check with your doctor before getting back into the swim.

JOGGING

This has become one of the most popular forms of exercise. Rain, shine, sleet or snow, joggers of all sizes and dimensions are out there doing their thing. If you feel you are ready to join them, you should be aware of some important points.

Jogging helps improve muscle tone and wind. It will firm up flab, but it won't perform reducing miracles. In fact, if you are still a little on the heavy side, jogging may cause muscle pulls if done too strenuously.

To avoid stress and strain on the knees and back, and foot problems too, stay off hard surfaces. The best place to jog is on a dirt surface, wearing proper jogging shoes.

If you are over thirty-five, however, be cautious. Don't start without your doctor's approval—and even then, start gradually. Begin with no more than a quarter-mile. Build slowly, by about an eighth-mile per day.

BALLET PRACTICE

Have you ever envied the firm muscles and fluid grace of a ballerina? Constant practice and rigid training developed her into the lovely creature who flits across the stage. While I can't promise you that practicing a few basic ballet exercises will lead to an engagement with the Ballet Russe, I can tell you they will help eliminate flab, tone your muscles, and add grace to your walk, to the way you sit, even to the way you stand.

To maintain balance in these exercises, it isn't necessary to install a practice bar. Hold on to the top of a chair, a table, or the top of your kitchen sink, leaving your legs room to swing easily.

Bends, or *pliés,* are warm-up exercises used by most dancers. Hold on to your chosen practice bar, plant your feet with heels together and toes pointed out. Keep your body straight and your fanny tucked in.

Now, bend your knees slowly, turn them out too, go

all the way down, and come up slowly. As you get closer to the floor, your heels will come up. Try to keep a smooth, even rhythm. Practice until you can rise without jerky movements. Background music in three-quarter time will help you get the feel of it.

Ballet kicks, or *battements,* which are excellent hip slimmers, are also practiced while holding to something for balance. The trick in doing these is to keep the knee of the kicking leg and the knee of the supporting leg straight at all times. If you kick too high, you may find it difficult to keep the supporting leg from bending, so ... kick lower. It is the action that counts. You aren't aiming for height.

Be sure you have plenty of room, stand with heels together, toes pointing out. With the outside leg, kick five times forward, five times to the side and five times back. Reverse and repeat with the other leg.

This next exercise is known as *port de bras,* which means movement of the arms, but it actually gives you a lot of movement over your body. Legs, arms, and waist all get a workout.

Hold on to your exercise bar, and remember to point your toes and keep knees straight. Now, arm above your head, swing the outside leg forward, not too high, and bend toward it. Then smoothly swing the leg back as you bend back. Leaving the leg back, bend forward. Finally, bring the leg into place to complete the set. Try to develop a smooth, flowing movement as you repeat: leg forward, bend; leg back, bend; forward, bend; swing the leg into place on the floor. Do a complete set at least three times with each leg.

"Very good," I can hear you saying. "Swimming, jogging, and ballet are great exercises. But let's face it, I haven't the time or patience. I'd hate having to get dressed and undressed three times a week. Besides, I'm *really* too busy to take out all that time."

If that's your problem, then you might find the following approaches more appealing.

EXERCISING AT YOUR DESK

Middle-age spread has nothing to do with age. It is an occupational hazard that eventually gets everyone who sits at a desk through most of the day and doesn't get enough exercise.

When you were younger, sitting at a desk in school didn't cause muscles to soften and weaken because before and after school you were always busy running somewhere. Always on the go, it never occurred to you that you were exercising.

Lack of exercise has caused the natural girdle formed by your abdominal muscles to weaken and spread. Don't let it keep spreading! Even while sitting at your desk, you can condition yourself with a minimum of effort.

Don't slump at your desk. Slumping cuts off oxygen and crowds vital organs, causes fat to collect at the back of your neck, and contributes to a bulky waistline. When you catch yourself slumping, lift your shoulders and neck, straighten your back, and suck in those abdominal muscles.

While sitting straight with muscles tightened, take the opportunity to do a few other exercises. Slowly touch your left ear to your left shoulder. Now the right ear to the right shoulder. Then raise both shoulders at the same time, getting them as close to your ears as possible. Then drop them way down.

You can exercise neck and shoulder muscles all day by remembering to turn only your head, not your body, when you look out the window, or toward the filing cabinet, or whatever.

Legs take the worst beating if you work in an office, because they were meant to be used, not stuck in cramped positions under desks all day.

To pep up the circulation in your legs, skip the elevator if you only have to go up or down a floor or two. And during the day, while at your desk, take a few minutes out for this exercise:

Sit straight at your desk. Under the desk, raise one leg straight out from the knee. Arch the instep and rotate your ankle until you feel the muscles pull in back of the knee. Do this with each leg separately, then both legs together. This is a good one to remember on long plane trips when your legs begin to ache because of the cramped space between the seats.

If you can't take advantage of the breaststroke because you don't swim, try this one at your desk. It is excellent for firming and developing chest muscles and firming flabby arms.

Just place both hands under the desk palms up, then push up hard, as though you were trying to lift the desk off the floor. Push harder, until you feel the energy coursing up your arms and across your chest. Stay that way as long as possible, then relax. Repeat it at frequent intervals.

EXERCISING AROUND THE HOUSE

Every exercise recommended for all-day desk sitters is also good for housewives. While sitting at your kitchen table rotating your ankles or working at firming your bustline, remember to sit up straight. No slumping!

Don't be lazy around the house. Walk as much as you can, using a good brisk stride. And suck in your stomach muscles.

While standing at your ironing board or preparing

dinner at kitchen counters, keep practicing the stomach-muscle squeeze. Tighten the muscles when you suck them in. Try to hold for a count of seven or eight without breathing. Then relax slowly.

And while doing housework, never, never stoop over to pick up things, to open drawers, or while dusting lower shelves. Bend at the knees and keep your back straight. You'll be avoiding back troubles while giving your knees and thighs a workout.

When walking around the house, get the habit of taking knee-high strides instead of ordinary steps. Throw those knees way, *way* up, creating a pull on your buttocks.

Are you hanging pictures, dusting, or performing any other tasks near the wall? Stop for a moment, place your hands flat against the wall, and step back until your arms are perfectly straight. Now slowly move your body toward the wall until your head touches, then move back. Do as many of these push-ups as you comfortably can—and repeat the process throughout the day.

Any mop or broom handle can easily be converted into an arm slimmer. Simply hold it horizontal in front of you, at shoulder level, palms downward. Keeping a firm grip and without lowering the handle, rotate it just by manipulating the hands and wrists.

Whenever you hold a can or a book weighing two or more pounds, take advantage of the opportunity. Fold your knees and bend slightly at the waist. Dangle the weight loosely in one hand. Now, swing that arm out and upward, allowing your torso to follow naturally in the same direction. Let the arm drop loosely, and repeat five times. Do the same with the other arm. By performing this exercise often, you'll find yourself instinctively increasing the number of arm swings, with resulting benefits to your waist and bustline.

Taking a shower? After drying yourself, still naked, stretch the towel in front of you, hip high. Walk forward by stepping over the towel. Bend only as much as necessary to maintain balance. In this manner, go about ten feet, and gradually increase the distance each time. Within a few weeks, your hips and thighs will start to show their appreciation.

As you can see, your home offers many opportunities for brief, regular, beneficial exercises. And once you become exercise-conscious around the house, you'll start concocting a few of your own.

The innovations are endless. For example, Marilyn Margulis, the eminent New York beauty instructress, teaches her class a new wrinkle in weight-lifting:

Fill a sock or stocking with dried lima beans, lentils, or legumes. Bring it to desired weight, tie tightly, and presto—you have a homemade dumbbell! As your arms' strength increases, you can keep raising the weight of this simple but effective exercise tool.

See how easily ideas can come? The following two categories, strictly speaking, are not exercises. Nevertheless, because of their growing popularity, they must be evaluated.

YOGA

For a while, doing yoga exercises as a means of gaining or maintaining a good figure was almost as popular as jogging. Perhaps because it carries a certain mystique.

Yoga is complicated. There are several points to consider if you're thinking of joining a yoga class. While the average class teaches simplified forms of basic exercises, ideally they should be individually adapted for each student, and for very good reasons.

Even in its simpler form, yoga requires a great deal of twisting and turning to attain correct positions. Twisting, turning, and straining can be downright dangerous for adult backs. Without proper supervision, what should have been a pleasant exercise session can easily lead to a chiropractor's office. Exercise is important, but it should be done sensibly and chosen carefully.

SALONS

Television and newspaper advertisements featuring svelte young ladies and handsome, muscular men are constantly luring customers into figure salons. For people who feel they need the discipline, this kind of regimentation will work. For a while, anyway. Until the novelty wears off and the entire procedure becomes tedious and tiresome. Remember, to derive any benefits from exercising you've got to enjoy it. It's no good if it becomes a chore.

Exercise salons stress the use of machines, some of which are totally useless. The machine bounces you around, and instead of exercise, you acquire a few black and blue marks.

The only useful exercise machine is one that makes you work against resistance. Here again, as with yoga, the machine should be individualized for you, otherwise it can be dangerous. The woman using it a half-hour ago may have been larger and heavier, with a lot more power in, say, her arms. Then you come along and try to work against that same resistance and—look out. You've pulled a muscle or, worse, slipped a disc.

Which brings us back to what I've been saying. Exercise, performed sensibly and carefully, will tone and lighten your body. Done in your chosen time and according to your needs, it can be fun.

Now, before doing our spot-reducing exercises, let's limber up.

BREATHING AND STRETCHING

Correct breathing strengthens your diaphragm and helps rid the body of inhaled poisons. When doing your exercises, don't tense up and hold your breath. Practice inhaling through your nose when you start a movement and exhaling strongly at the finish. Try to become conscious of your breathing.

If you feel tired and out-of-sorts during the day, find a quiet corner, stand straight with arms at your sides, and inhale deeply. Then exhale through your mouth loudly, so you can hear it. Exhale, exhale, exhale. You'll be surprised how refreshed you will feel.

Before you begin your morning exercises, while still in bed, start the day off with a little conscious breathing and some stretching to limber you up for your exercises. Inhale—one, two, three, four. Exhale—one, two, three, four. Now, still lying there, stretch your legs luxuriously, like a cat, until you feel the back of your knees pull.

Get out of bed slowly, still stretching. Stand with your feet apart, arms up over your head, and reach for the ceiling with each arm alternately. Keep them both up and reach left, reach right, reach left, reach right, as high as you possibly can without moving your hips. Do this ten times with each arm.

Now you are ready for the exercises that can help you from your neck to your ankles. All can do something for you. Work at them easily and daily. Don't overdo. Don't expect miracles overnight.

NECK

1. Position yourself flat on your back on the bed, head and neck hanging over the edge. Let your head hang low so you feel your neck muscles pull. Hold this position for about a minute, then slowly raise your head and neck as straight up as you can, keeping your shoulders flat on the bed. Work up to three of these neck pulls a day. But be careful. You are working toward a firm, attractive neck, not a stiff one.

2. Lean your head way back, then start to roll it around in a complete circle. Slowly to the side, forward toward your chest, side, and way back. Keep your neck limp and pretend it has no bones. Work up to about five or six neck rolls daily.

3. Sitting straight on bed or chair, try to touch your chin to your chest. Come up slowly and try to touch your head to each shoulder. Count slowly ... chin and up, left shoulder and up, right shoulder and up. Repeat five times.

SHOULDERS, ARMS, AND BUSTLINE

1. Start by raising your elbows to your bustline and touching fingertips in front of you. Swing elbows hard, as if they are going to meet behind you. Feel the pull in your shoulders? Back to first position and repeat ten times.

2. Holding your arms straight at your sides, lift your shoulders as high as you can. Don't move your neck,

just your shoulders. Let shoulders fall back to normal position and repeat ten times.

3. Stand straight, expand your chest, arms straight out to each side. Now rotate arms in a circle from front to back. Count to twelve, then reverse the circle and rotate arms from back to front for a count of twelve.

4. Sitting on the floor, legs out straight, chest high, extend your arms as far as possible in front of you. Then do the breaststroke. Turn palms out and swing arms in an arc behind you, bend elbows as you bring arms forward and back to first position. Do this about eight times, and really move so you feel the pull in your chest, arms, and shoulders.

5. Bend elbows and clasp fingers tightly in front of you. Push palms hard against each other, then pull and try to separate your fingers. If you do this correctly, you will feel the pull on underarms and pectoral muscles. Repeat five times.

6. Even if you hate swimming, you may enjoy this "fish-out-of-water" exercise. It requires a narrow surface like a piano stool or coffee table. Place your belly comfortably across the width, elevate your legs—and swim! Keep those legs up—rotate your head and neck in rhythm with the arm movements. It doesn't have to be fast—just comfortable. Time is what counts—increase it gradually.

MIDRIFF, WAIST, AND STOMACH

1. Stand straight, feet together, keeping legs rigid. Bend from the waist—first to the left side, then to the right. As you move, raise your hands up to your armpits in a pumping motion, in rhythm with each side bend. Do this eight times. This one is great for preventing the spare tire around your midriff.

2. To avoid putting too much pressure on the lower back, do your toe-touching exercises while sitting down. Sit with legs apart, stomach in. Relax your knees and stretch arms out. Bend forward with right hand trying to touch left foot. Don't strain. Bend only as far as you can. Repeat with left hand trying for right foot, and continue five times each side.

3. To firm stomach muscles, lie on your back, raise both legs slowly and straight up, until they are at a right angle to your body. Keep toes pointed. Bring legs toward your head as far as possible, then lower them Repeat five times.

4. Lie on your back with both knees tucked up to the chest. Holding hands clasped around knees, roll forward into a sitting position. Hold your back straight and head up. Then slump (here slumping is permissible) and roll down again. Repeat five times.

5. Lie flat on your belly, elbows out, one hand atop the other. Rest your chin on your hand. Keep your legs stiff, toes extended. Slowly elevate your chest (including the arms) and legs (at the hip) all at the same time. Hold at the topmost position for a second or two, then slowly return to prone. Build to fifteen times per session.

6. The old-fashioned bicycle movement is still one of the best exercises for flattening tummies. Remember how it is done? Lie on your back with hands supporting your hips, lift your legs high, pretend you are riding a bicycle, and pedal away. Maintain a slow, circular movement, keeping legs high until they are tired. Relax a few minutes, then repeat. Increase the frequency each day.

HIPS, THIGHS, AND BUTTOCKS

1. One of the most effective hip and buttock reducers is what I call the "derrière bounce." Sit on the floor

with legs stretched out in front of you. Fold your arms across your chest so you won't be tempted to use them for support. Then simply wriggle across the room on your derrière by shifting from side to side. Five times daily and you'll be amazed at the results.

2. Lie on your back with legs straight out and arms stretched out at your shoulders. Pull legs up with knees bent, then swing knees first to the right until thighs touch the floor, then to the left. Keep shoulders and arms flat to the floor. Roll from side to side rapidly so thighs actually slap the floor. Start with five a day and work up to ten.

3. Again lying on your back, raise one leg at a right angle to your body and lower slowly to the floor. Keep toes pointed and leg rigid. Repeat five times, then change to the other leg, resting between the changeover. Try to increase to about twelve times with each leg.

4. Off your back this time, and onto your hands and knees. Keep arms straight. Raise one knee and bend your head to meet it. Now, swinging your leg back and up, raise your head and arch your back. Do this five times with each leg.

5. Stand with hands on hips. Lift one knee as high as possible, then slowly extend it behind you. As your leg naturally tends downward, your task is to keep it moving as slowly as possible. Start with five times for each leg, gradually increasing to fifteen.

6. Sit in a soft seat, preferably a couch or easy chair. Extend your arms loosely to the front or side. Try to stand up without lowering your arms. If this one seems "impossible," train yourself by performing the same movement on a firm seat. Eventually you'll "graduate" to the softer chair, where you should strive for a minimum of ten stand-ups per session.

7. Lie down on your left side, keeping your body straight, left arm under head, right hand placed in front for balance. Raise the right leg as high as possible, then

lower it slowly. Repeat for a total of ten times. Roll over and do the same with the left leg.

KNEES, LEGS, AND ANKLES

1. To shape up chubby knees, sit straight in a chair and stretch one leg in front of you with toes pointed. Stretch hard and hold for a count of five. Repeat with the other leg, then with both legs at the same time. Hold on to the chair seat for support so you will find it easier to sit straight.

2. Stand with legs together and arms stretched out to the sides. Swing one leg up at an angle and bring opposite hand to meet it. Reverse to the other leg and hand. Try to keep in constant motion, with no hesitation between swings. Start with five times on each leg and try to achieve eight to ten swings.

3. Holding the back of the chair with your right hand, grab your left instep with your left hand. Now, pull your leg back. Repeat three times, relaxing the leg between pulls. Reverse and do the same with the other leg.

4. Hold on to a chair back and rise up on your toes. Press your knees together and do a deep bend, staying up on your toes all the time. Move your knees slowly from side to side, trying not to move your hips. Repeat at least six times.

5. An excellent leg shaper-upper is to stand with your toes on a thick telephone book with heels on the floor. Rise on your toes, then drop heels back to the floor. Repeat ten to twelve times.

6. Stand about a foot from a wall and lean into the wall with your stomach. Keep heels flat on the floor. Hold for about half a minute, then relax and repeat three more times.

7. And last but not the least. For shapelier ankles, practice these old dance steps whenever you get the chance. Move across a room sideways, first bringing your toes together, then your heels, then toes, then heels, and so on until you are out the door.

This survey of head-to-toe spot-reducing movements is designed to give you a variety of choice. Determine the part or parts of you that need slimming or firming. Then pick the exercises most suitable and enjoyable. One or two from each category is sufficient, provided you maintain regularity—a *minimum* of three times a week.

Remember, however, that spot reducing is not a substitute for the total exercise program. To keep your youth and loveliness—to maintain your vibrance, vitality, and sexual vigor—your entire body needs constant maintenance.

Chapter XVIII

A BEAUTIFUL, EASY WAY TO SLIM DOWN

Don't you believe that fat is beautiful. It isn't!

Imagine what you could accomplish if you had a "secret weapon"—an "elixir"—which, in combination with easy exercise, would hasten safe weight loss and heighten your beauty potential.

Am I about to prescribe a new miracle drug? Hardly. This "elixir" is nothing more than a combination of three basic foods: honey, oil, and vinegar—we call it the "HOV" formula.

HOV works where other diet plans have failed, because it makes you feel dynamic, cheerful, and well-fed—instead of tired, irritable, and half-starved.

HOV can add years of vigorous health and happiness to your life, as well as put you at the peak of your beauty potential.

HOV improves dry, prematurely wrinkled skin by helping it maintain its own moisture balance.

HOV not only removes those ugly extra pounds; it also redistributes your weight in better proportion by helping to break down unwanted fat deposits in your arteries and in the sedimentary portions of your body (abdomen, hips, buttocks, upper thighs).

Honey, safflower oil, and apple-cider vinegar can help you rid yourself of that undesirable "excess baggage" you could never seem to budge with exercise. Each healthful, helpful component of this unique formula has a specific job to do. In combination, they provide you with that necessary energy and feeling of well-being that rigid calorie-counting diets lack.

HOV gives you a beauty boost *while* you slim down to a desirable size. You don't have to wait for weeks to feel satisfied. This "magic triad" is safe, economical, and effective.

The "HOV" Formula

2 teaspoons honey
2 teaspoons safflower oil
2 tablespoons apple-cider vinegar (must be apple-cider vinegar)

Mix well. Take 3 times daily, ½ hour before mealtime or as otherwise directed.*

Taken regularly, the HOV formula helps you lose weight slowly, steadily, and reasonably, without hunger pangs, flabby skin, or jittery nerves.

* The quantity above is for a "single dose." If more convenient, you may make up to a 3-day supply, keeping it refrigerated. In using "HOV," you may consider a whiskey jiggerful as being about the proper amount for a single dose, although more may be taken if desired.

A tall order for such a small package—but it works. And there's no high price tag on this method. *Honey, oil, and apple-cider vinegar* can be bought in many supermarkets and in all health-food stores. To be slim and svelte, you need only determination and HOV.

The HOV formula, used in combination with a high-protein, low-carbohydrate diet, will recondition your body into using unattractive stored fat for fuel instead of relying on carbohydrates for ready energy. You will actually begin melting your unwanted body fat and converting it into energy.

To accomplish this, you will of course have to cut down your intake of the ready-fuel foods: sugar, starches, and alcohol (the beauty banishers). When the supply of starches and sugars diminishes, your body will be forced to use up the fat it stored away for energy. The honey in HOV, however, will provide you with all the ready energy you need, so you will not feel tired and hungry during this reconditioning period.

Here's how HOV works from within.

Pure *honey* is the ideal appetite appeaser. Aside from being rich in important minerals, some B vitamins and C, it is the best source of quick energy.

By consuming two teaspoons of honey (in HOV) a half-hour before your regular mealtime, you will not feel starved, you will eat slower and not as much. This modification of your eating behavior leads to better control of what you eat.

Natural honey, used in moderation since it is a concentrated sweetener, is the best appetite suppressant there is. This 99 percent predigested natural sugar immediately enters your bloodstream and appeases the hunger signal set off by the hypothalamus gland. Taken a half-hour before a meal, it regenerates your energy level and relieves your gnawing craving for food. And since honey is readily utilized by the body for energy, it isn't applied directly to your hips—the way many candy-bar calories are, for example.

The second ingredient of the "big three" in HOV is safflower oil. This pure, natural, unsaturated oil provides you with necessary dietary fat (which is *not* fattening). And you do need some fat to maintain silky skin, fight wrinkles, and add sheen to the hair. Fat supports the kidneys and other organs, insulates you for warmth and protects your skin.

Of all the vegetable oils, safflower oil provides the highest amount of the fatty acids necessary for life. It also helps prevent water retention in the tissues. It helps your body to change sugar to fat more slowly.

As a fat, it prevents hunger pangs by allowing food to digest more slowly in the stomach. For that reason, this wonder oil keeps you feeling well-fed on less food—and that's the goal of every slender-minded woman, isn't it?

Without sufficient fat in your diet, the fat-soluble vitamins (A, D, E, and K)—and an important digestive enzyme, lipase, are inhibited. This can lead to a breakdown in the orderly way the body governs itself.

A fat-deficiency runs parallel with many vitamin deficiencies. So you must supply the body furnace with necessary fats. But they must be *unsaturated* fats—(those that are soft or liquid at room temperature. Safflower oil is probably the best source of these vital beauty fats.)

Aside from its obvious health benefits, safflower oil elevates your beauty level: it gives your skin glow and your hair gloss. Adding this oil to the diet often dramatically improves eczema and dry, flaky skin. Such a simple thing—but what a difference! You look good, feel good. And all the while this uncomplicated little oil is working away at dispelling fat deposits and, as an extra bonus, smoothing your skin.

The third item of the terrific triad—HOV—is naturally

fermented apple-cider vinegar, and it *must* be apple-cider vinegar, usually available in health-food stores.

As a beauty booster, cider vinegar helps melt away layers of fat—in much the same way it would dissolve a pearl (which is really solidified fatty oyster exudations). It does the job of banishing the blubber you've built up over a period of time.

The cider vinegar in HOV works "undercover" to rid your tissues of ugly lumps and bumps that have been dumped there. The HOV formula allows you to reduce with the confidence that you will look and feel marvelous *as* you become more slender, more attractive.

For even better health results while on HOV, take 50 mg. of vitamin B-6 *twice daily*—for a total of 100 mg. per day. Because when fat is burned for energy, water is produced in the body. Vitamin B-6 regulates abnormal water storage and eliminates bloating.

For optimal results, be sure to take HOV before every meal. It must be working in your system when you sit down to eat.

If, on occasion, you can't take your premeasured HOV with you, don't despair. There are many ways to take honey, oil, and vinegar.

Honey in *herb tea* is delicious. (Regular tea contains caffeine and acids; acids cause hunger.) And you can have vinegar and oil as salad dressing.

HOV helps regulate your "appestat," the automatic weight-regulating mechanism in the hypothalamus that adjusts your appetite to meet your energy requirements.

The normal stomach triggers a "full" feeling to the brain when adequate food has been ingested. The unfortunate thing about this nerve mechanism is that it does not function as swiftly as most of our other nerve impulses. It's a little on the lazy side, and a certain amount of time must elapse before the "full" nerve has a chance to signal the brain.

Therefore by eating too rapidly it is easy to consume about 30 percent more food than you really need or desire before the stomach's "full" nerve can send the message to the brain.

But by eating more slowly, chewing foods thoroughly, and allowing a couple of minutes to elapse between meal courses, the "full" nerve will have time to function sooner ... and, of course, this results in your eating about one-third less food per meal and still feel fully satisfied.

Your appetite (the *desire* for food) often dictates how much you eat instead of your hunger (the actual *need* for food). To get it back in line, you must restructure your eating attitudes and habits. This, in turn, will remodel your body into better proportions.

Dr. Richard B. Stuart, a specialist in the control of obesity, states that you must become *aware* of your eating behavior before you can modify or change it. He advocates record-keeping for this purpose.

Every time you eat *anything*, list what you ate, what time it was, where you ate it, in whose presence, and how you felt when you decided to eat. WHAT, WHEN, WHERE, WHY.

After a week or so, you will be able to look back and establish a regular eating pattern. You may discover that loneliness or anger triggered your urge to eat—or that you tend to indulge when you feel unloved or bored. You may find that you use visitors as an excuse to wolf down more than your usual share of goodies.

Once you realize your pattern, you must work to overcome the temptation to eat under those circumstances. It helps to understand why some people are "trapped" into obesity.

According to Dr. Judith Rodin, an associate professor at Yale University and a researcher in the field of obesity, there is no one single factor which causes obesity, but a series of several factors.

First, overweight people often have higher baseline insulin levels (which speeds the conversion of sugar into fat) and enlarged fat cells (which enhance fat storage). This means that the fatter you are, the more likely you will continue to gain weight unless you break the chain.

Secondly, being heavy promotes physical inactivity, which causes fewer calories to be burned.

Unhappiness is the third force that keeps people fat. The social stigma of being fat causes them to attempt to diet, but when they are frustrated by the prospect of failure (cheating on a diet) they start to overeat again, which makes the vicious circle continue.

You can condition yourself not to associate movies with candy bars and popcorn, television with snacks. You could begin by drinking a glass of water (even with a dash of lemon juice) whenever you feel the "munchies" coming on (except before mealtime, when you would take HOV). Water helps flush out accumulated wastes and 6–8 glassfuls a day are beneficial.

HOW TO EAT TO LOSE WEIGHT

1. Take HOV (Honey, Oil and Vinegar) half an hour before each meal.
2. Eat foods high in protein—lean meats, fish, fowl, low-fat cheese, eggs, sunflower seeds, soybean foods.
3. Never skip any of the three basic meals—especially breakfast. Late risers and light workers can do well with only two meals per day.

4. Eat slowly—insalivate food to help digestion. Chew very thoroughly.
5. Cut down on salt—it causes water retention in the tissues. But do drink 6–8 glassfuls of water every day.
6. Cut down on animal fats—the less you eat of them, the better. And that goes for all goods that have animal fats.
7. You're better off without it, but if you *must* eat bread, limit yourself to two slices per day.
8. Avoid the terrible trio of refined sugar, white flour, and mixed drinks. Not only are they fat makers—they are also "sugar makers."
9. Avoid highly seasoned food that stimulates the appetite.
10. Take daily a complete vitamin-mineral supplement (Nutri-Time is recommended), extra vitamin C (at least 500 mg.), and other vitamin supplements as needed.

COOKING AND PREPARING TO LOSE WEIGHT

1. Broil, grill, bake, or roast meat and poultry.
2. Broil grill, bake, or poach fish.
3. Boil, poach, or scramble eggs.
4. Avoid fried foods whenever possible.
5. Lightly steam vegetables—keep them crunchy to satisfy your "crunch craze."
6. Trim all fat off meat, preferably before you start cooking it.
7. Eat *water-packed* tuna and salmon. (If water-packed is not available, drain and wash oil off the regular commercial varieties—which are usually less expensive than the dietetic, or water-packed, products).

8. Prepare meals so there won't be any leftovers—always leave the table slightly hungry.
9. Use small plates instead of dinner plates. This will make portions appear larger.
10. Avoid all convenience foods—TV dinners, pretzels, potato chips. And never eat while watching television. This association leads to unnecessary snacking.

There is mixed evidence about how much of a problem fat cells are. "If you were fat as a child under five, it in no way dooms you to a lifetime of fatness," says Dr. Richard B. Stuart.

So you shouldn't feel because you were a chubby cherub, you are destined to remain a portly person. Self-image has a lot to do with keeping any weight loss permanent. You should not think of yourself as "formerly fat," but as slender and normal at last!

Temptations are the biggest setback for any dieter. You have to learn how to handle any enticement that may cross your path. You'll never reach your goal of a sleek shape if you reach for the wrong foods whenever you have the urge to nibble.

HOW TO HANDLE TEMPTATIONS

1. Never go shopping for food when you're hungry.
2. Eliminate all the cake mixes, brownie mixes, and other snacks from your pantry shelves.
3. Hang the most unattractive, heaviest picture of yourself on the refrigerator door along with a picture of a beautiful, slim model.
4. Weigh yourself each week on the same scale, in the same clothes, at the same time of day. Then post

the weight in large block numbers on the kitchen cupboards.

5. Never eat when overtired or upset—just to fill the void. Sip water and lemon juice instead.
6. In a restaurant, decide what you want, then order before the others. Ask for a salad immediately (with oil and vinegar). Don't let the breadbasket sit in front of you.
7. While out socially, should someone urge you to "go off" your diet, acknowledge their positive motives and ask them to help you stick to your diet.
8. Write reminders to drink 6–8 glassfuls of water on all the mirrors of the house.
9. Don't cave in completely if you do cheat and sneak a cookie. One transgression doesn't make you an all-out failure, and doesn't make the rest of your effort meaningless. If you are put in a situation where you feel you *must* eat to be polite, half a portion is plenty! Take an equal number of calories away from your next day's menu.

Reshaping your eating behavior and your meal content means reshaping *you*. With the terrific triad of HOV at your service, you'll discover that slimming becomes easier than you had thought possible.

You can and you will win the fight against fat with a beauty boost from HOV. You can scale down to a lightweight and be a knockout yourself! After all, they say dynamite comes in a small package!

The beauty boosters—honey, oil, and vinegar—can knock out the beauty banishers—white sugar, white flour, and hard fats.

And YOU are the winner!

More beautiful and more slender than ever.

Chapter XIX

THE SEVEN-DAY HOV DIET FOR BEAUTIFUL SLIMMING

The suggestions listed below are, of course, subject to change—depending on availability, individual taste, and budget. In adapting them for your own use, just be guided by the *types* of food, making whatever changes suit your preference. All you do is to take it from there.

EVERY DAY

Before each meal
The HOV Formula—see previous chapter for instructions. Take not less than a jiggerful (about 1 ounce) before each meal.

After breakfast and after dinner
Vitamin-mineral supplement (my choice is Nutri-Time)

Extra vitamin C (at least 500 mgs)
Other vitamins and supplements as required

Sometime during the day
1 tablespoon lecithin granules and 1 teaspoon brewer's yeast (powder or flakes) stirred into bouillon, tomato juice, or skim milk, or sprinkled on salad or in food.

Important
Drink a minimum of 6 glassfuls of water each day—8 is better.

ANYTIME

Midmorning, midafternoon, or whenever desired
Cup of consommé, bouillon, or instant vegetable broth—hot, jellied, or on the rocks.
Buttermilk, skim milk, or yogurt (up to a pint a day total intake)
Coffee and tea—especially herb teas, decaffeinated coffee, or coffee substitute (no cream or sugar, but a little skim milk may be used if desired)
Choice of Eat-All-You-Want Foods and Snacks listed at end of this chapter

FIRST DAY

Breakfast
½ grapefruit

Scrambled eggs (cooked in lightly oiled pan or double boiler)
Choice of beverage

Luncheon
Baked or broiled fish (with parsley, optional)
Lettuce, celery, cucumber, and watercress salad, with HOV as dressing
Glass of skim milk or buttermilk

Dinner
Lean roast beef
Shredded cabbage, carrot, and bean-sprout salad
Asparagus
Fresh pear or apple
Choice of beverage

SECOND DAY

Breakfast
1 medium orange
6–8 oz. plain yogurt with 2 tsp. bran flakes
Choice of beverage

Luncheon
Broiled hamburger with slice of tomato and onion
Shredded cabbage salad with HOV as dressing
Glass of skim milk or buttermilk

Dinner
Crabmeat cocktail

Chicken, broiled or grilled (remove and discard skin)
Broccoli
Leafy-green salad with HOV as dressing
Honeydew and watermelon balls (if in season. If not, a small apple)
Choice of beverage

THIRD DAY

Breakfast
½ small cantaloupe or grapefruit
2 heaping tbsp. cottage cheese topped with yogurt
Coffee Slim (⅔ cup coffee and ⅓ hot skim milk)

Luncheon
Small tin tuna (drain off oil)
Celery, radishes, and raw cauliflowerettes
Fresh seasonal fruit
Choice of beverage

Dinner
Broiled liver with mushrooms
Steamed carrots, minted, if to your taste
Mixed green salad with HOV as dressing
⅔ cup of diced pineapple—fresh, if in season. If not, use canned with natural juices.
Choice of beverage

FOURTH DAY

Breakfast

Fresh strawberries or sliced orange moistened with orange juice

Grilled cheese open sandwich (made by spreading 2 oz. cheddar cheese on slice of whole-grain bread. Place under broiler for a few minutes to melt cheese.)

Choice of beverage

Luncheon

2 all-beef frankfurters

Cucumber, sliced beet, and chicory salad with HOV as dressing

Glass of buttermilk

Dinner

Patty made with 4 oz. ground veal mixed with 1 tsp. raw bran flakes. Broil or grill to desired done-ness

Combination salad with HOV as dressing

1 ripe banana

Choice of beverage

FIFTH DAY

Breakfast

½ grapefruit

Cheese omelette (2 eggs, 1 oz. cheese)

Choice of beverage

Luncheon
Small tin of salmon, drained
Raw carrot, cucumber, and zucchini sticks
1 apple or pear
Glass of skim milk or buttermilk

Dinner
Broiled or grilled fish (red snapper, if available)
Steamed cauliflower or cabbage
Mixed green salad with HOV as dressing
Slice of melon or fresh fruit
Choice of beverage

SIXTH DAY

Breakfast
Whole orange, peeled and sliced
Salmon patty made with 1 tsp. bran flakes
Choice of beverage

Luncheon
Shrimp, 5 or 6 medium size
Green bean, celery, and onion-ring salad
Glass of skim milk or buttermilk

Dinner
Lamb shanks, small to medium
Steamed shredded turnips
Tomato and watercress salad with HOV as dressing
Wedge of cheese and ½ sliced apple
Choice of beverage

SEVENTH DAY

Breakfast

½ grapefruit

Chicken-liver two-egg omelette. Or one slice whole-grain bread with ⅓ cup cottage cheese. Put under broiler for a few minutes to slightly brown cheese.

Choice of beverage

Luncheon

Tomato bouillon (⅔ cup of bouillon made with cube and ⅓ cup hot tomato juice)

Chef's salad with seafood, dressing of your choice

Choice of beverage

Dinner

Broiled steak

Mushrooms, grilled or broiled

Romaine, shredded raw spinach, and sliced radish salad with HOV as dressing

Fresh or frozen raspberries (or other berries) topped with 1 tbs. yogurt

Choice of beverage

The green and combination salads in the diet above can be as varied as the seasons, so no recipes are given for them. Make them to suit your individual taste by combining several of your favorites from the following low-carbohydrate list:

Leafy Greens and Raw Vegetables for Salads

Lettuce, romaine, endive (curly and French), escarole, chicory, young raw spinach, mustard-spinach, dandelion, mustard and turnip greens, lamb's-quarters, sorrel, bean sprouts, tampala, watercress, chopped parsley, celery, cucumber, cabbage (green, red, Savoy and Chinese), green and red peppers, scallions, radishes, leeks, onion rings, tomatoes, shredded or sliced young beets, carrots, turnips, zucchini, summer squash, broccoli, cauliflower, sliced raw mushrooms, eggplant, and pimiento strips.

Next to protein, the leafy greens are probably a dieter's best friend. They're high in vitamins and minerals and the lowest of all vegetables in carbohydrates, so try to have them often, either alone or mixed with other raw vegetables. And if you haven't taken your formula HOV before eating, don't forget to mix it into your salad as a dressing.

Just a reminder: without HOV you might be tempted to overeat, especially fattening, high-carbohydrate foods.

EAT ALL YOU WANT—OF THESE FOODS

Group I

Vegetables, Raw or Cooked

artichokes, globe and Jerusalem
asparagus
bamboo shoots
beans, green and wax
green and red pepper
kale
lettuce
mushrooms
mustard greens

bean sprouts
beet greens
broccoli
cabbage
cauliflower
celery
chard
chicory
Chinese cabbage
Chinese water chestnuts
cucumber
endive
escarole
parsley
pickles
pimientos
radishes
romaine
sauerkraut, low salt, naturally fermented
spinach
summer squash
tampala
turnip greens
watercress
zucchini

For slimming snacks to stave off hunger, keep your refrigerator stocked with eat-all-you-want vegetables and prepare a day's supply at a time. Wash and dry them in a clean tea towel, save some for cooking or for dinner salads if you like, cut the rest into bite-sized pieces, and refrigerate them in a bowl covered with plastic wrap. They'll stay crisp, fresh, and ready for nibbling whenever you are.

LET YOURSELF GO WITH SEASONINGS

Group II

Herbs, Spices, Seeds, and Sauces

You may use any of these as freely as your taste dictates:

Cider vinegar, lemon juice, horseradish, mustard, and soy sauce.

Caraway, celery, dill, poppy, and sesame seeds.

All herbs, fresh and dried.

Almost all spices, including curry, paprika, and freshly ground black pepper *

* If you are acne-prone, avoid all "blushing seasonings" so as not to make the condition worse.

Chapter XX

TENSION AND STRESS—THE BEAUTY BANDITS

Whenever the subject of beauty arises, the conversation invariably turns to the realm of fashion modeling. My work as a nutritional counselor frequently brings me into that world, where I have had occasion to observe, close up, photographers at work with their models.

Those sleek, sensuous young ladies are indeed a pleasure to behold—not only because of their loveliness, but also because of their professional poise and charm. Yet watching them also saddens me, because I know that most of them will be forced to seek new careers by the time they are in their thirties.

Why this inevitability? Why does a model's beauty fade so fast, even though she diets and exercises faithfully?

Much of the answer lies in the life she is forced to lead. Pounding the pavements in her fiercely competitive field, the average model rarely knows where her next dollar is coming from. Financial worries combine with an unending fear that she may already be past her prime.

Battered by these pressures and anxieties, she is in a constant state of turmoil. Her blood pressure rises—she sleeps poorly—her digestion and metabolism are askew. Small wonder that despite all the physical care she gives herself, frown lines and mouth creases appear at an early age, while her skin loses its radiance and texture. After a while, not even the photographer's touch-ups can mask all the blemishes.

Tension and stress are often referred to as "bandits" of beauty. I think "sneak thieves" would be a more accurate description. To understand why, find your biggest mirror and take a good look at yourself. Don't smile or strike a pose. Just stand there and look.

Is it a pleasant, relaxed face you see? Or are there frown lines, creases, and a tight mouth? Does the face in the mirror appear tense and drawn? Have the stresses and strains of everyday living begun to leave their mark? There's a good chance they have, without your ever realizing it.

Check around as you travel to work or on a shopping trip. Notice the unrelaxed faces showing signs of tension, stress, and inner conflict.

How does your face look to other people?

"Aging," says Dr. Hans Selye, noted authority on the subject, "is the sum total of all the scars left by the stress of life. He points out that these "scars" not only cause lined faces, but also dried skin, thinning hair, brittle fingernails, and a host of other symptoms associated with waning youth.

To understand why, let's take a brief look at the culprit.

Simply put, stress is the subjecting of our minds and

bodies to situations or conditions which they are not fully equipped to handle.

Stress results from emotional entanglements—such as love, hate, grief, jealousy. It can come from the pressures of day-to-day, people-to-people involvements or from environmental pressures. Most of the time, you have little awareness that you are experiencing a stressful condition.

When the body is under stress, certain parts demand extra nourishment. Like machines operating above normal capacity, stiffened muscles and jangled nerves require excessive energy to keep from breaking down. All that energy must come from someplace, and that place is the body itself.

Swiftly depleted of its normal reserves, the body must seek energy from its own protein sources, usually the lean-meat tissues that constitute our organs. Thus deprived of their nourishment, all organs—including the skin—begin to malfunction and eventually deteriorate.

All of us are subject to a certain amount of stress from today's fast living pace. This we cannot do much about. But most of the stress we undergo—up to 90 percent—can be eliminated with some forethought and preplanning.

The trouble is, many people accept the growing number of lines on their face, and even mental conflicts, as a necessary part of living. To them tension and stress have become a way of life.

For instance, are you the person who sets the alarm for 7:00 A.M. and then waits until the very last minute to get out of bed? Then is it rush, rush, rush to get out of the house and to work? Often with only a cup of coffee to hold you until lunchtime?

Or does this sound like you? The woman who always gets tangled up at breakfast time because you get up late and the kids are waiting for their lunchboxes? Your husband waiting for his coffee? You can't believe the day has just started.

Or are you the type who lets things work on you quietly?

Say your husband has suddenly called to announce he's bringing an important client home for dinner. You're completely unprepared, and you know the pressure you'll be under for the next few hours. But instead of objecting, you fume in silence.

Or you are the loyal, hardworking secretary whose boss saves an entire week's dictation for Friday afternoon? Do you ever voice a complaint? Or do you wind up muttering to yourself while you type furiously, under enormous pressure?

Dozens of incidents like these, ranging from major to minor, happen all day. You may even think you thrive on this kind of tension, but sooner or later it must take its toll.

Somewhere in there you may say, "It gives me a pain in the neck," or, "I think I am getting a headache." But that's not the end of it. For these are the situations that lead to the lines on your face—the chemical and mental "scars" that Dr. Selye described.

You may even be one of that group known as "workaholics," people so obsessed with work that they can't ever seem to stop, at the office or at home. Tension and stress are their constant companions, because they never find time to rest or relax. Driving yourself relentlessly is a sure road to depression and illness, which leave their marks on your face.

To be sure, it's not only your protein balance that suffers. Stress also burns up vitamin C, which your body needs to strengthen skin cells and tissues. Vitamin A, so essential because it aids in preventing dry, rough skin, is used up rapidly under even the mildest tension.

"All right," you say, "tension and stress are ruining my looks. But what am I supposed to do about it?"

The answer can be summed up in one word: RELAX.

"Relax! You must be putting me on," you say.

One of the commonest questions I hear is, "Don't you think I've tried relaxing—a thousand different ways?" Yet somehow relief for many seems barely adequate and wears off quite soon.

There are a number of misconceptions about relaxation. The greatest one is that all you have to do is lean back, close your eyes, say, "I'm relaxing," and that will do the trick.

At best, such relaxation is of limited value. It simply postpones the tensions while you take a breather. It does not expel them. As soon as you un-relax, the pressures mount rapidly.

Going to movies, reading, listening to music are all fine and fulfilling forms of relaxation. But if yours is a severe stress, these solutions are all too temporary, because they're not available often enough.

Relaxation is something of an art. Each of you must seek and perfect the forms that work best for you. They needn't be complicated—only specific. Specific for you.

One of the loveliest women I know tells me that whenever she feels tension and hostility mounting, she goes for vigorous exercise—especially a long, brisk walk.

I know many people who don't wait for their tension to surface. They take time out for five or ten minutes, whenever they can, to lean back, close their eyes, empty their minds of problems, and think of only their favorite things—skiing, swimming, lying in their lovers' arms, to mention a few.

A tension-ridden executive whose efficiency I admire, says she does it by shutting out the world for a few minutes and letting the words and music of a favorite song drift through her mind.

"After a few minutes of that," she told me," I ask myself what am I doing trying to carry the weight of the world on my shoulders."

Another friend "drops out" by spending an hour daily, right in her office, reviewing her Spanish lessons. "I'm learning Spanish," she said, "because it stimulates my mind and takes me away from the daily grind."

When tension starts to mount, it frequently sends out warning signs to key parts of the body. The following simple routines can sometimes nip stress in the bud:

1. Place your hands against the back of your head and press your thumbs gently into the base of your skull. Hold for as long as possible—do not pulsate or massage.
2. While resting your fingers on your forehead, gently ease your thumbs under the earlobes. Again, do not move thumbs or fingers. Just hold.
3. Place your hands behind your neck so your fingertips touch the nape. Massage gently—very gently—for thirty seconds, then rest for thirty seconds. Continue this alternating procedure for a total of five minutes.
4. Reach behind you, resting your clenched fists against the small of your back. Massage and rest, as in number 3 above, for five minutes.

Unlike figure- and face-beautifying exercises, the best anti-stress techniques are those that can be performed anytime you feel the need. If one that you do at home is impossible to do at work, your relaxation is only half-effective. Unless, of course, you have a different procedure for each place.

Discussing your tensions with others can sometimes bring beneficial results. For one thing, it's a relief just to get them off your chest. Then, too, you meet people with similar problems, who might join you in convenient remedies.

Some years ago a physician retained me as a consultant to help him discover the causes of so much stress and tension suffered by many of his patients who worked in one of the large advertising agencies.

Among others, I talked to a lovely secretary whose stress showed in many ways. By the end of the day she was a bundle of nerves, unfit to enjoy the evening ahead. Others in the secretarial pool had similar tendencies to tension. We learned that some of these women, like the secretary, enjoyed playing bridge. This led to a daily bridge tournament at lunchtime.

It was enough to eliminate the young secretary's stress problem. That period of concentrated relaxation helped to wind her down for the rest of the workday.

Which brings to mind one of the most fallacious forms of relaxation from the work routine: the coffee break. Maybe sitting down and sipping the hot liquid has a momentary tranquilizing effect. But beware when that caffeine goes to work on your nervous system! That's when you'll *really* need to relax.

If you feel you *must* drink something during a break, make it warm soup or fruit juice. But even better, try a brisk walk around the block. It not only relieves tension; it also provides exercise to firm up your figure.

For people who enjoy exercising often and have the time for more extensive tension remedies, this next one has proved effective in many cases:

1. Slowly bend or stiffen your right foot. Relax. Then your right calf. Relax. Next, your right thigh. Relax.
2. Repeat with the other leg. Maintain the relaxation throughout the entire session.
3. Tense your abdomen. Relax.
4. Tense and relax each arm, in sections, as you did your legs, hand, upper arm, forearm.
5. Tense and relax the lung area. Breathe deeply several times.

6. Tense and relax your shoulders. Drop them.
7. Tense your neck. Circle your head several times, rotating first to one side, then the other. Drop your chin to your chest. This is one area where most people are tense.

This next series, deceptively simple, has produced some remarkable results:

1. Select a quiet room and sit in a comfortable chair. Adjust yourself so you are as relaxed as possible. This will probably mean slouching forward a bit, resting your hands on your thighs, and keeping your feet flat on the ground, somewhat in front of the position of your knees.
2. Close your eyes. Now, consciously relax all your muscles, beginning with the feet. Move up through your legs, your stomach, your chest, your arms, your neck, and even your face, jaws, and mouth. When your jaw muscles are really relaxed, your lower teeth will probably not be touching your uppers.
3. Breathe through your nose and draw the breath into your belly, which should be rising and falling. Become aware of your breathing, but don't take deep breaths. They aren't necessary. Breathe normally and naturally.

Now, as you breathe out, think of a single word and say it to yourself. Inhale. Exhale and repeat the word.

Keep your muscles relaxed and continue breathing rhythmically, easily, in and out, repeating the word with every exhalation.

Continue for 10 to 20 minutes. When you finish, sit quietly for a while and then gradually open your eyes.

Generally, it has been found that the best way to relieve a tension is to replace it with another tension. Not another devastating pressure that will add to your woes, but a healthy, enjoyable tension which drives out the negative one.

The excitement of a sports event is one such tension. No one is more tense than a pair of chess players—and no one is more relaxed when the match is over. The tension of rolling for a strike at the bowling alley is only a prelude to the feeling of well-being that follows.

Active relaxation, in general, seems to be more effective than passive forms. Perhaps that's why women with hobbies, with active interests outside the home or office, seem to retain their beauty longer. Or haven't you noticed?

Whatever activities you choose, it is also desirable to counteract tension by supplementing your diet with the vitamins which tension destroys: A and C. Extra benefits might be gained from the nerve-calming B-complex.

A ONE-DAY STRESS CURE

And when it comes to planning active relaxation, what can be more relaxing than the very acting of making yourself lovely?

I'm not referring to occasional minutes snatched each day for applying makeup or performing exercises. Nor do I mean a few weekly hours at the hairdresser's or a sauna.

For complete, beautifying relaxation, how about a long, luxurious stretch of time—say a whole day or even a weekend—when you do nothing except pamper yourself?

"Impossible," you say? Saddled with family or work obligations—or both—how could you find time for such indulgences? Besides, even if the time were available, who could afford it?

You'd be surprised at how easily (and inexpensively)

you can luxuriate in the total relaxation of your own "self-made spa." All it takes is some imagination and a little pre-planning.

Have a schedule ready in advance. Not an ordinary workaday schedule, mind you, but a full-time "pampering plan." Load it with pleasant activities—especially those which you enjoy doing all by yourself.

In order to achieve the best results, you'll need complete privacy. Remember, your object is a delightful, unashamed way of self-indulgence, free from family cares or work problems.

It's a day, for example, when you can soak in a scented tub for an hour or more, with no one to knock on the bathroom door. It's a day when you can try a new facial or learn another exercise without the kids staring and giggling at you.

Perhaps Grandma, Dad, or a friend can take the children out for the day. If that's not possible, make arrangements for a sitter to come in so you can get out. Borrow a friend's apartment, or check into a local motel. The idea is to give yourself a tension-free spirit-lifting day of beauty.

Even if you've been on a slimming diet for weeks—maybe months—this is the day to select menus with extra taste appeal, your favorite foods. Pre-cook and, if necessary, freeze them so you won't be wasting precious time in the kitchen. On the other hand, set the table as if you were serving royalty—because today you *are* the queen.

Make everything easy for yourself. Assemble beforehand any ingredients of the energy cocktail or natural beauty aids you plan to try. Shopping is "illegal" on this special day.

Television is off-limits, as well as any mind-cluttering activities like coffee klatsches or telephone conversations. This is your very private, very special day—so make the most of it. Discourage any visiting. Take the phone off the hook.

Channel all your energy into beautifying experiences. Feed your skin, your body, your mind and ego with all the alluring benefits you can muster.

Free your face from makeup, let it breathe. But do indulge it in a special mask while you enjoy a mind-resting repose in the tub or posture-chair.

Or start your day with a stimulating, brisk walk, smiling all the while. When you come home, settle into gardening, painting, embroidering—or whatever your favorite hobby happens to be. If reading is your thing, this could be your opportunity to bone up on the latest beauty information.

Spend your entire day totally absorbed in your own well-being, pampering yourself, without a care in the world. It's the most complete and thorough relaxation you can give yourself—a one-day stress cure that lasts indefinitely.

And as you come to the end of this glorious, stimulating day, start planning your next one, whether it be a week or a month later. Just thinking about it will relax your features in a warm, glamorous slow.

By no means should you postpone that day until you sense the "pressures" building.

The time to tackle stress is before you feel it. For it may be lurking sneakily, insidiously draining your skin of its radiant hue while carving your first crowfoot.

Don't wait for tension to strike. Begin now to find your best anti-stress, pro-beauty weapon.

Chapter XXI

ARE YOU MISSING YOUR BEAUTY SLEEP?

Though it seems a far cry from the subject of this book, I would like you to think for a moment about cats. That's right, ordinary cats—like your household pet, perhaps, or the ones prowling your neighborhood.

Have you ever noticed how often a cat washes itself, never satisfied until its fur is smooth and sleek? Have you ever watched a cat manicuring its claws, cleaning its eyes, trimming its tail? Many zoologists believe that cats are the world's most beauty-conscious creatures.

Now, look at yourself. Like an alluring pussycat, you bathe, manicure, and trim. You eat only the foods your body requires—in just the right quantity—and you give yourself a daily quota of slimming exercises.

Yet something is not right. Despite assiduous self-care, after many years, your eyes may be starting to wrinkle and grow puffy. Cracks are forming at the corners of your mouth. Breasts have begun to droop;

your belly going to pot. Unlike the cat, your beauty seems to be fading with age.

What could you be doing wrong? Once again, I commend your attention to that original "glamour-puss"—the cat.

Observe a few cats' sleeping habits, and you'll discover that no two are identical. You'll notice how cats, when they do sleep, curl up, relax completely, and close out the world around them. If they're restless at night, they get up and do something useful for themselves. If they feel weary during the day, they quickly retreat into their proverbial cat naps. And when they awaken, it is with a lusty yawn and a graceful, unlimbering stretch—signs of healthful sleep.

Yes, there's much that beauty-oriented women can glean from our feline friends. And maybe all you need to learn to complete your beauty program is a proper approach to sleep.

Is it possible, for example, that you haven't been getting the right kind of sleep?

Notice I didn't say the right *amount*. I said the right *kind*. Eight hours, six, four . . . it hardly matters. If you spend the night tossing fitfully, breathing poorly, waking frequently—then you are not sleeping well, no matter how many hours it lasts.

And nothing can destroy a lovely complexion as quickly as a bad night's sleep. It leaves you mentally numb, with tired eyes, dulled complexion, and low spirits—phenomena which add nothing to a woman's charm.

The more restfully you sleep, the more efficiently your mind and body replenish their energy during that period. Deny them this chance to renew energy, and they won't function properly. Along with the telltale signs that show on your face, your body will become listless, your muscles and posture will sag, your mind will feel dull.

"True beauty sleep," says Dr. Richard J. Wyatt of the National Institute of Mental Health, "can vary from three hours a night to eleven or twelve."

A short, deep sleep does you far more good than a long, disturbed one. If you wake up feeling restored, you've had enough sleep no matter how many hours it lasted. Eight hours filled with restlessness can still leave you tired, with eyes and face that show your fatigue. The amount of sleep needed to relieve fatigue and restore energy varies according to age, the degree of fatigue, the state of your nerves, and your all-around health.

What, then, is insomnia? Does such an illness really exist, or is it "all in the mind"?

Actually, insomnia is a true clinical condition caused by certain diseases or psychological disorders. A severe case of chronic insomnia—complete deprivation of sleep—is obvious to any of its victims. Its physical and mental devastations are so apparent you don't need any expert to tell you about their beauty-robbing potential.

What we're concerned with here is the more subtle form of insomnia. Insomnia which you may not even realize you have. Insomnia which doesn't keep you wide-awake, yet sneakily intrudes on your slumber. Insomnia which prevents beauty sleep.

To cope with such forms of sleeplessness, you must ferret out the primary causes. What are they?

Worry. If you go to bed with your mind full of business or household problems and keep turning them over in your head, your worrying will easily keep you from sound sleep. Add to that your worry about not falling asleep and you're really in trouble.

Bedtime is not the hour to plan tomorrow's work schedule. When the brain is stimulated, you remain awake. The best remedy is to acquire the habit of mental relaxation.

Reading at bedtime has always been a good way to relax. But it should be light reading, possibly even dull—better yet, boring! The more boring the reading matter, the sooner you will find your eyes getting heavy. Try the telephone book for dull reading. Nothing could be duller!

A brisk walk before bedtime is an excellent way to relax. And a warm bath just before delving into that dull book will easily cut your reading time by two or three pages.

Muscle-tension. After a strenuous day of tennis or a concerted effort at housecleaning, you may not feel a thing—until bedtime. Your mind may be relaxed, but the aches and tightness in your muscles will conspire to keep you awake.

To get rid of those aches, get right back out of bed and try the following exercises:

BEAUTY-SLEEP STRETCH

Stand with your feet apart, rise on your toes, and stretch your arms straight up high over your head. Reach for the ceiling. Then start loosening up and let every part of you go limp, starting with your arms, until you are bent over and drooping toward the floor. Repeat this about three times.

BEAUTY-SLEEP BEND

Lie on your back on the floor. Bend your legs and bring knees toward your chest. Lie there relaxed for about five minutes.

If you're sleeping with your mate, remember that just

about *the* best bedtime relaxer is sex. Almost every muscle in your body is brought into play during this "exercise." Aside from the pleasure you derive, you will be performing isometric exercises in concert. And what can be more relaxing afterward than to fall asleep nestled in the arms of your loved one?

Poor eating habits. Because the body takes two or three hours to digest a meal, late-night eating causes your metabolic machinery to work overtime when it should be closing shop for the night.

Give yourself a good four or five hours between your final meal and bedtime. And avoid starches and sugars—the carbohydrate foods. They can keep your stomach churning all through the night.

On the other hand, don't go to sleep hungry either. Hunger is a common sleep thief among dieting women.

If you feel the need for a bedtime snack, a glass of skim milk or buttermilk is enough to set the digestive processes into light, brief action, drawing blood from your brain and muscles to relax them even more. And milk, particularly buttermilk, contains calcium and lactic acid, two nutrients that nourish the sleep center of the brain. Yogurt is another excellent pre-bedtime snack.

Other sleep-inducing nightcaps are: peppermint tea (a natural relaxant). Lettuce soup (a mild sedative). Or a tablespoon of honey mixed with hot water and lemon juice.

Booze and pills. Alcohol, if you drink enough of it, seems to put you to sleep. But liquor, like coffee, is basically a stimulant and may reverse the sleep process. Then your beauty sleep is turned into restless, sometimes fitful slumber.

Sleeping pills run a similar pattern in the brain, with the added risk of dulling your mind and reflexes all through the ensuing day. This leaves you even more tired at night, tempting you to increase your dosage.

Which is another way of saying: booze and pills are dangerously habit-forming.

Wrong schedule. Beauty-*less* sleep can sometimes be traced to the fact that you do your work at the wrong time of day, fighting your biological time clock. Some people are day-oriented, some are night-oriented.

Body temperature rises and falls about two degrees through each 24-hour period, dropping to its lowest point from two to six in the morning. As you become more active, body temperature rises. You are at your highest point, mentally and physically, when your body temperature reaches its peak.

If by early afternoon you really get going, really begin to sink your teeth into whatever you are doing, you are a day person. Conversely, if your body literally doesn't warm up until late afternoon or early evening, you are more of a night person, who might function better in a life-style that lets you sleep later in the morning.

Whatever may cause your problem, it is important to remember that there are no hard-and-fast rules to achieve proper sleep. For sleep to make you more lovely, it is only necessary that you recognize your unique, individual needs, tailor your schedule to fit those needs, and stick to the schedule.

Many people, for instance, find that they can relieve sleep-inhibiting tensions at night by the simple expedient of napping during the day.

These lucky persons, who have the ability to fall asleep wherever and whenever they wish, use their 20- or 30-minute catnap as a refresher and restorer. For them the nap is a quick way to escape from the pressures of the world. And since a short nap consists of the first and deepest sleep, they may actually save about an hour of nighttime sleep.

Every woman needs some trick, some way through which she stops trying to cope for a while—some way to "turn off," to relax and refresh mind and body.

But not all of us have the time or the make-up for a daytime nap. Many have discovered that a nap makes them lethargic and interferes with their ability to fall asleep at night.

If you are a non-napper, you may find one or more of the following suggestions will help you relax away daytime tensions:

1. Whenever you are on the phone, lean back, close your eyes, and relax your muscles. This will be easier to do at home, but try it at work as well.
2. If you do some traveling on your job, take advantage of every moment waiting for planes and trains; close your eyes and sink into repose.
3. Close your office door, put your feet up on the desk, and think of anything but business for ten minutes.
4. When you feel tension mounting, take a few deep breaths and let them out quickly, as if you were sighing. As you expel each breath, you will feel muscles let go all the way to your feet.
5. Sink into a comfortable chair, let your head drop back, stretch out your legs, lift your arms, drop them limply at your sides, and relax all your muscles.

Now, let me ask you a very important question. Have you taken a close look at your bed lately? A good bed, which contributes to restful sleep, is not a mere luxury. It is a necessity.

During normal sleep, we change positions thirty or forty times a night. A good bed is one wide enough and long enough to allow for this movement, while providing even support.

When you go to bed, are you lying *on* the bed or *in* it?

If when you lie down, all the body's vital points—neck, trunk, pelvis, and legs—are supported, that's a good bed. If the bed is hard in some places, soft in others, if you sink into it and your spine curves, it's a bad bed and you should do something about it. Buy a new mattress, or add a bed-board between mattress and spring to firm up the one you have been sleeping on.

Next, take a look at your pillow. If it is a big, thick one, get rid of it. Thick pillows interfere with circulation in the head, while helping to create neck wrinkles and double chins. Using them encourages you to sleep with your face in strange positions. You press your face into the pillow and twist your neck.

Continually lying on your face can cause muscles to flatten and facial contours to change. Check your mirror tomorrow morning. Are there signs of creases and folds in your face? If you see any, your oversized pillow may be the cause.

The best way to sleep is with no pillow at all. Still, if you feel you *must* have one, it should be a pillow small enough to tuck neatly under your neck. If you don't have one, make a tight roll out of a bath towel and use it under the back of your neck to keep neck and chin in a firm but comfortable position.

As for correct bedwear—it should be kept to a minimum. Sleeping in the "raw," though not considered esthetic, is actually the healthiest way to sleep. Each time you move during normal sleep, you rustle the covers enough to allow fresh air to caress the pores of your skin and help them breathe. That's far more comforting and healthful than the confinement of pajamas or long gowns.

The "baby-doll" or "shortie" type of nightgown is the closest approach to the healthy minimum that one should wear to bed. Someday designers will come up with exactly the right brief style of sleepwear, probably based on bathing suits or ballet costumes—esthetic, healthful, and comfortable.

A good bed, tension-relaxing exercises, and comfortable sleepwear all help you to restful beauty sleep. But is the environment of your bedroom doing dreadful things to the skin of your face?

There's a good chance that, unless you sleep in a damp basement night after night, your face is being robbed of essential moisture, because the atmosphere is drier than you are.

To overcome this problem, cosmetics manufacturers once advised using night creams that were supposed to *nourish* the skin. Now these are called old-fashioned by the same manufacturers. This year's night creams offer *protection,* with so-called "unique" formulas that block out air and seal in moisture.

Unquestionably, your face should get added moisture while you sleep, to keep your skin wrinkle-free and young-looking. But not necessarily with a high-priced, dubious formula, packed in a jar that costs more than the cream.

To complete preparations for beauty sleep, pat your face gently with a safe, sane, and sensibly priced moisturizer. Then you will be all set for pleasant dreams.

There is nothing magical or mystical about sleep. An occasional bad night should never be cause for concern. Even full-scale insomnia once in a while is harmless. And chances are when you think you've been up all night, you've actually dozed off more frequently than you realize.

Still, if you simply can't overcome that wide-awake feeling, you're better off taking advantage of it rather than trying to fight it. Leave the bed and relax with some easy reading or restful music. Perhaps you can use the opportunity to complete some house chores or office work.

Most of all, don't agitate over it. The body easily makes up for infrequent moments of wakefulness.

So don't let sleep frighten you. Be like the graceful, alluring pussycat: Make sleep work for you . . . to keep you beautiful.

Chapter XXII

WHAT'S BEAUTY WITHOUT ENERGY?

You can have the face of an angel and the most voluptuous body imaginable—but without energy, you're just another lifeless rag doll.

And who wants to be a pretty package with no contents? An empty shell that people find boring?

Energy is a positive way of life. It means power, vitality, enthusiasm. It's the life force that motivates every man and woman to strive for the heights. Utilizing your total energy, you can accomplish your "Impossible Dream" . . . improve your personality . . . introduce excitement into your life . . . become more beautiful.

Every woman dreams of being loved and cherished. Do you have what it takes to attract and *keep* a man? If not, you'd better sit down and evaluate your problem. Perhaps the following simple test may help you.

What are your honest answers to these questions:

Are you sleeping a lot longer than you once did?
Do you skip meals?

Has your weight crept up and you're not doing anything about it?

Are you sloppy about your appearance?

Do you eat candy bars for energy?

Has your husband or lover stopped complimenting you?

If your answer is "yes" to even one of these questions—dear lady, you're in the middle of a personal energy crisis! And you'd better dig yourself out of that pit of lethargy—fast!

It really *is* possible to conquer your deadbeat feeling, to realize your fullest beauty potential, and to capture (or recapture) the missing romance in your life. But you have to work at it. If your DREAM factor is out of kilter, you must correct it.

Energy is a complete plan. It is the only means by which we can attain our goals.

Physical energy gives you the capacity to do anything.

Mental energy gives you the motivation to accomplish anything.

Emotional energy gives you the ability to love what you are doing with your life.

Energy is the force that brings out the hidden beauty within you. Its magnetic quality attracts men to you. It promises amorous fulfillment. Without energy, sex can fall flat—if, indeed, it ever gets started!

Energy is the secret of so many of our successful women. "Successful" because they have fulfilled their dreams, whether those dreams were of family or of fame.

Energy was the secret that made Eleanor Roosevelt a great humanitarian.

A combination of energy, brains, and determination

got Ella T. Grasso elected governor of the state of Connecticut.

Endless energy was the secret that made Grandma Moses a successful artist at the age of ninety.

Energy was the source of more than a hundred mystery novels by British writer Dame Agatha Christie.

One of the world's outstandingly beautiful women, Imelda Romualdez Marcos of the Philippines, is also a dynamo. Her abundant energy has been channeled into beautifying her country and helping her people—with the result that the city of Manila has become the showplace of the Orient. Mrs. Marcos also rations some of her energy to the maintenance of her beauty—something every woman has an obligation to do.

Energy can make *you* more beautiful, more interesting, more fulfilled—and change your entire outlook on your daily living. It radiates through your face, your voice, your touch. Men instantly notice a woman who brims with vitality. She has a special talent for enjoying life. She's in harmony with herself and a pleasure to be with.

Energy and perseverance can achieve almost any goal. A dynamic woman can set the world—or her man's heart—on fire. Her energy affects those around her.

What must you do to awaken the "other woman" inside you?

Begin by thinking of yourself as an original Work of Art. You can perfect any portion of yourself by repainting or resculpting. You can learn to change negative attitudes about yourself. You just have to know the method.

You should realize it's not just one particular thing that makes you feel as if you're stagnating, that your sex appeal has dried up and many of your interests have evaporated.

Your energy stream is fed by several "underground springs"—diet, rest, exercise, attitudes, and maximum maintenance. Each influences the others, and all are necessary for a super-energized you.

Here is the wonderful fact: you are capable of channeling your energy into whatever avenue you choose. Toward a more beautiful skin. A more satisfying sex life. Or toward becoming a more totally beautiful woman.

But to accomplish this miracle, you've got to destroy your old lazy ways. How? Quite simple really. Here is your five-point plan of attack:

Remember those "underground springs" I mentioned earlier? They form the DREAM factor that can make your dream come true—a new dynamic YOU.

D-R-E-A-M is the key to all energy. It is a positive five-step plan to attain maximum energy output.

D—A DIET of foods *high* in protein and *low* in sugars and starches builds energy.

R—REST fortifies energy. Sound sleep and relaxation refresh your brain and your body.

E—EXERCISE begets energy. It builds up your energy level.

A—ATTITUDES channel energy. Your attitudes gauge your mental outlook on life. How you interact with other people. What you think of yourself.

M—MAXIMUM MAINTENANCE keeps energy at its peak. It charges up the body's battery and changes you into a ball of fire.

The high protein-low carbohydrate diet will help in your quest for abundant energy. But there are specific energy foods I want you to have. And so I have created the VITALITY BEAUTY COCKTAIL to make sure you really get set in high gear.

This dynamo of a drink is not a meal replacement; it is a peak-performance potion. Some even say it works as a "love potion"—but if it does, consider that a plus factor! Its power works from the inside out. It taps a secret vein, and what you discover is as good as gold: High Energy!

VITALITY BEAUTY COCKTAIL

Thoroughly mix the following ingredients:

- 4 oz. (half glassful) fresh milk—preferably skim milk. (If fresh milk is not available, add 1 tbsp. skim milk powder to 4 oz. water and stir thoroughly to make a "reconstituted" milk.
- 1 oz. pineapple juice (unsweetened)
- 1 tsp. desiccated liver powder
- 1 tbsp. honey
- 1 tbsp. black molasses (also known as treacle)
- 1 tsp. wheat-germ oil
- 1½ tsp. lecithin granules
- ½ tsp. kelp powder

Take this twice daily *for one month*—once, shortly after arising—again about an hour before dinner or as a late-afternoon snack. After that, for maintenance, once daily upon rising will suffice to keep you feeling more vibrant, more alive.

A word of caution: don't swallow in gulps. Sip slowly; insalivate before swallowing.

This delicious cocktail will convert that "pooped out" feeling to "pepped up" spirit. And a lively, spirited woman is one who attracts a man's attention. Once you develop the energy habit, you won't ever want to slip back into your old ways.

If you aren't already taking vitamin-mineral supplements, I do hope you will start now. Vitamins and minerals are really important for maximum maintenance of your precious body.

Modern life brings on stress. So most people need a little extra help to feel their best. A really complete vitamin-mineral supplement that I personally use is called Nutri-Time. You may wish to look into it for your own use; most health-food stores sell it. Where *your* health and *your* energy are concerned, prevention pays one hundredfold!

As your DREAM factor gets into shape, you will no longer feel undernourished, unfulfilled, and unloved. Instead, you will be creatively alive. Things will happen because you'll have the energy to make them happen.

Your man will be fascinated by and enjoy the great improvements in your appearance, your temper, your ego. He will notice how much better you feel—how much more alert and alive you are!

Improving your DREAM factor will make you a more beautiful person with abundant energy to realize your own dreams.

You may find it hard to believe that energy can change your way of life—but it will. For one thing, your sex life will improve. And don't think your husband or lover won't sit up and take notice. Your man will be delighted with the change in you.

Who would have thought that just eating different foods—and drinking that power-packed Vitality Beauty Cocktail—would make such a big difference? ENERGY is behind it all—backing up your effort to accomplish your heart's desire, to bring out the radiance of beauty within you.

Some other rewards to which an energy-charged person can look:

You'll be more open-hearted, see people in a light that shines beyond your own problems. As an example: a nasty store clerk will never again upset you. Your new calm will help you understand that the clerk's attitude is probably due to dealing with so many versions of your *former* self.

Energy now surging through you will invigorate you to do more exercises. Pretty soon your body slims down to shapely proportions.

And a further reward: your man will begin to follow you around the house with lovemaking on his mind! And *that* will help channel your new found energy where it belongs! Can you think of anything more delightful?

Once the dormant energy within you gets into high gear, you will grow more beautiful every day. Your eyes will sparkle. Your skin will glow. The warmth of your smile will be *felt* for miles. You won't just talk about realizing your dreams anymore, you'll do it!

With energy—you just can't miss.

Chapter XXIII

BEAUTY AND SEX— THE PERFECT PARTNERSHIP

Some ten to fifteen years ago, the world—and America in particular—was caught up in a swirl of sexual liberation. This era, subsequently dubbed "the sexual revolution," has brought about many changes.

Sex has become less and less "taboo" in the movies. TV talk shows are rife with panelists, from famous actresses to everyday housewives, baring their deepest intimacies. And there is an unending stream of sex manuals which graphically describe the many exciting variations.

I am not about to comment on the merits of this new wave. Nor do I wish to enter another opus in the "how-to" market. I leave these tasks to sociologists and psychologists.

From my viewpoint, however, there is one pleasing fact that emerges from the manuals and discussions—a fact I have stressed for nearly fifty years, namely: *sex is one of nature's best beauty aids.*

Find that hard to swallow? Then let's see what happens when two lovers "get it all together."

To start with they *communicate*—through their talk, their touch, their actions. Like musical instruments, their bodies reach a crescendo in movement and burst into a rousing climax.

Throughout this foreplay and build-up, it is not only your sex glands that are aroused. Every square inch of your body is stimulated. Exercise is imparted to all your muscles. You breathe more deeply, inhaling more oxygen, expelling more wastes. Blood courses to every cell—even in the skin—providing life-sustaining and life-renewing nutrition.

Even without a partner, sex can achieve the same beautifying results—sometimes more so. Sexologists have long recognized that by stimulating and arousing themselves, many women are able to extend the length of their orgasms, thus achieving greater health and beauty benefits.

And what are some of these benefits?

With or without a partner, prolonged, passionate orgasm extends the period of isometric exercise for the entire body. This helps to break down fatty tissue and tone up muscles.

Each awakened body organ works a little harder, causing you to perspire more freely. Your pores exude trapped wastes which can cause dryness, rashes, and other blemishes.

A sexually stimulated heart can temporarily elevate blood pressure by as much as 20 percent. It sends a rush of blood to the skin surface, sometimes even creating a brief, reddish rash. Nearly all sexually aroused women exhibit this sex flush on occasion.

It is a healthy sign. For the flush means that more fresh blood is reaching the body's surface, nourishing and renewing the skin, hair, and nails. A beauty treatment from the inside—and what a pleasure to give or receive!

Warm, wonderful sex tenses many muscles which control movement. This accounts for the strong contractions in the neck, abdomen, and face (especially around the mouth). As orgasm approaches, the hands experience involuntary clutching, clawing and grasping, which contribute to shapeliness as I pointed out in another chapter.

Sex is one of the most effective tension relievers and sleep inducers. Never forget: stress and insomnia are two of the worst enemies of beauty. Stress leaves you with wrinkles, frown lines and poor appetite, all of which reduce your beauty potential.

Insomnia can be a source of dark circles under the eyes, poor skin tone, dull hair, and lethargy. You certainly won't look beautiful if you can hardly keep your eyes open!

Though not a strenuous exercise, sexual intercourse burns up about 200 calories. Substitute a little loving every morning, instead of ten minutes of regular exercise, and you will continue to work off unwanted weight—the fun way!

Of course, sex by itself is not going to improve any woman's loveliness. Without proper nutrition, the health and beauty benefits of intercourse are minimized. In fact, without the full range of vital nutriments you may find your sexual energy itself on the wane.

A full high-protein breakfast of scrambled eggs with cheese added, whole-grain toast, whole fruit instead of juice, bran served with low-fat milk, and beverage provides the fuel to recharge your body. It may mean getting up a half-hour or so earlier. But isn't this "sacrifice" worth the deeper contentment it brings to your love and sex lives?

Bear in mind, too, some of the foods that help keep

the sex organs in peak condition: egg yolks, garlic, honey, low-fat milk, almonds, filberts, sunflower seeds, pumpkin seeds, wheat germ, and yogurt.

When making love, good hygiene is important for achieving a complete, beneficial sex act. No woman who offends the masculine nose or eye can be truly desirable. Cleanliness is tantamount to beauty.

To bring out your best beauty, cleanse your entire body (especially private parts) thoroughly at least once a day. Don't just mask body odors with perfume—use soap and water to wash off the putrefying wastes that seep through the pores and harden on your skin.

Special attention should be paid to cleansing the genitals. Gently clean inside the creases and folds of the vulva and outer lips with a mild (not a deodorant) soap, using your hand. Dragging a nubby washcloth over the area may irritate, even injure, the sensitive tissues on which your enjoyment of sex depends.

Douching is not necessary for the health of your sex organs. In fact, some of the chemicals in commercial douche preparations, such as carbolic acid, can be quite abrasive on this tender area and may cause allergic reactions.

Femininity, the touchstone of loveliness, is also an integral part of sex appeal. It means something different to each person, but in general it is a vision of a desirable, fragrant female body—one that is well-groomed and attractive.

To achieve this effect, don't adopt an unflattering fashion simply because it's "in." Stick to clothes that do something for you and you alone. Men like soft, revealing lines which let their imaginations run rampant.

Every lover has his preference. If your man loves legs, show yours. Don't hide them under slacks or jeans, day in and day out. If he's partial to breasts, wear close-fitting tops with scoop necklines or tantalizing semitransparent blouses. You don't have to be big-breasted to be beautiful and sexy; just know what to do with the equipment you have.

Once you have the musts for sex appeal, you may still have to confront and conquer hang-ups which interfere with reaching a total climax. Even in these days of sexual frankness, there are a surprisingly large number of women who go through life without ever experiencing orgasm.

The reasons are many and varied. But nearly always it's mental interference that prevents orgasm, not physical incompatibility. If that is your problem, some professional counseling might provide the solution.

Beauty and sex appeal are still one of the best combinations going. Each complements the other. Each contributes to the total fulfillment of lovemaking.

A healthy mind and a body bursting with beauty—shaped by good nutrition and exercise—are the best sexual stimulus you can share with your man. Relax and let the orgasm sweep you into a deeper dimension of beauty.

Chapter XXIV

YOUR DAILY BEAUTY PLAN
(A Personalized, Individual Program)

And so you are ready to begin.

You have read all the "hows," the "whys," and the "wherefores" of natural beauty. Now it is time to put those principles into practice in an easy, organized, painless fashion.

There is one lament I hear often during my lectures and consultations. It goes something like this:

"So I've been eating the wrong foods–applying the wrong cosmetics–neglecting my exercises. But that's been my whole life. Can I change it overnight?"

My answer is always a hearty, emphatic YES!

Literally overnight, you can shuck all your bad beauty habits and adopt your new regimen without the slightest inconvenience. And though it may take you a while to *see* the results, chances are you'll start *feeling* the glorious difference after your very first day.

Of course, no two persons can stick to precisely the same schedule. Individual lives vary, and so must their programs. But whatever the variations, one fact is certain:

If you stick to your own daily, personalized beauty plan—with the right diet and the right attitude—you will be rushing down the road to super-loveliness. How can you go wrong if you persevere for perfection?

While avoiding bad habits, start cultivating the good habits of your individualized beauty routine. You can work out a suitable schedule patterned around your individual life-style and responsibilities.

Don't be wary or worried about the following sample beauty plan. It is the *ideal* for which to strive. To be effective, it *must* be flexible. What is most important is that it be regular.

As your lifelong beauty program becomes second nature, you will become more becoming. A beautiful new YOU will rise from the ashes of your old bad habits . . .

THIS IS THE FIRST DAY OF THE REST OF YOUR LIFE!

BEFORE GETTING UP: • Let your head hang over the edge of the bed for a few minutes to stimulate circulation. Count to 50 if you have time.

UPON ARISING: • If slimming, prepare and slowly imbibe HOV (refer to Chapter 18 for directions).

BEFORE BREAKFAST: • Begin the day with an acid-based soap-and-water wash-up, cleansing according to your skin type. First your hands, then your face.

- Follow facial cleansing with cider - vinegar - and - water toner, to restore acid mantle. Seal in the water on your damp skin, with the moisturizer of your choice.
- Protect and enhance your natural beauty with subtle application of hypoallergenic makeup (if you must use makeup) highlighting your best beauty features.
- Splash on your own special fragrance.
- Prepare and slowly drink the Vitality Cocktail (recipe in Chapter 22) while you prepare breakfast. Here's a suggestion:

BREAKFAST:

- Unsweetened orange juice, 1 or 2 eggs and/or whole-grain, unsugared cereal, herb tea, or decaffeinated coffee.

AFTER BREAKFAST:

- If a morning person, take your day's quota of vitamin-mineral supplements. Don't overlook Nutri-Time, for multiple protection; a minimum of 500 mg. vitamin C; 25,000 I.U. vitamin A; Lecithin granules; 400 I.U. vitamin E.
- If slimming, list what you have eaten in the food diary, to establish eating pat-

tern in order to change behavior.

MID-MORNING:

- Drink at least one glass of water.
- If hungry, enjoy a small protein snack.
- Apply sunblock or sunscreen with PABA if you will be out in the sun for an extended time.
- Open windows for fresh air.
- Exercise for 10 minutes. Try spot-reducing or office exercises (Chapter 17).

HALF-HOUR BEFORE LUNCH:

- If slimming, prepare and slowly imbibe HOV (recipe, Chapter 18).

LUNCH:

- Meat, (red and lean), fish, eggs or cheese; vegetables. mixed greens or lettuce and tomato salad; 1 slice of whole-grain bread; fresh fruit; herb tea, decaffeinated coffee, or skim milk.

AFTER LUNCH:

- If slimming, list luncheon menu in your food diary.

HALF-HOUR AFTER LUNCH:

- Drink a glass of water.

MID-AFTERNOON:

- Suck in stomach muscles 10 times while working.
- Lubricate face with vegetable oil or mayonnaise for 10 minutes.
- Exercise all 55 face and

	neck muscles, practicing movements outlined in Chapter 10.
	• Whistle while you work—a wonderful mouth exercise!
	• Drink a glass of water.
	• Give yourself an eye treatment (Chapter 13) and/or a face-lift with an invigorating mask, according to skin type (Chapter 6).
	• Catnap if necessary—and if possible.
	• If hungry, eat a high-protein snack.
HALF-HOUR BEFORE DINNER:	• If slimming, prepare and slowly imbibe HOV.
DINNER:	• Clear soup; green salad; large portion of lean meat, poultry, or fish; vegetables, lightly cooked.
	• Choice of one—potato or slice of bread; unsweetened dessert, (only if you must); herb tea, decaffeinated coffee, or skim milk.
AFTER DINNER:	• If slimming, list foods eaten in your diary.
	• Drink a glass of water.
EARLY EVENING:	• Limber up with bend-and-stretch exercises (Chapter 17).
	• Unwind while exercising through swimming, jogging, neck massaging, etc.

OR

- Enjoy a 20-minute brisk walk for easy exercise—you may meet and make new friends while seeing the local sights.

WHILE WATCHING TELEVISION:

- Remove shoes and practice foot exercises with bottle and/or tennis ball (Chapter 15).
- Drink a glass of water.
- Give yourself an acne treatment when necessary (consult Chapter 7 on blemished skin).
- Give yourself a gentle scalp massage.
- Read something light to induce sleepiness.
- If your feet ache, soak them (see Chapter 15 for suggestions).
- If hungry, have a high-protein snack—low-fat or cottage cheese; sunflower seeds.
- Instead of TV, you may wish to listen to quiet, restful music to wind down.
- Once a week, give yourself the beauty treat of a manicure followed by pedicure.

BEFORE BEDTIME:

- Enjoy a warm, scented bath or shower.
- Massage your arms and legs

to stimulate circulation and to achieve a lovely rosy hue.

- Shave legs, as necessary.
- Shampoo hair, as necessary.
- Use oil or conditioner (Chapter 12) on hair as necessary. If you color your curls, touch up as necessary.
- Set and dry hair.
- Brush hair to luster, then style it.
- Cleanse hands, neck, and then feet in a soapy basin.
- Remove makeup with cleanser.
- Apply cider-vinegar-and-water toner.
- Spray face with water from atomizer and apply moisturizer of your choice, very generously around eyes.
- Drink a glass of water.
- If a night person, take your vitamin-mineral and other supplements—according to your needs.
- Apply vegetable oil to fingernails and toes.
- Tip your eyelashes with castor oil.
- For better sleep, drink one of the relaxing beverages listed in Chapter 20.
- Reapply your own glorious fragrance for enticement.

As I said at the start, this daily schedule may be altered according to your needs and tastes. You might, for example, prefer to wash your hair and set it in the morning rather than at bedtime. Body and face exercises needn't be performed at the time of day specified. And some of the suggested treatments (such as for feet or eyes) are not necessary every day.

However you vary it, this healthful, beauty-full maintenance of your countenance and your curves is a solid investment for today—as well as for all of your tomorrows. You will leave the ranks of mediocrity and step into the elite circle of the Totally Beautiful Woman.

Chapter XXV

BEAUTY IS TIMELESS—IT KNOWS NO AGE

As you embark on your journey into loveliness, you've discovered ways to slim your waist and firm your torso, extend your lashes and trim your brows, highlight your cheekbones and subdue your wrinkles.

In short, you've learned the art of allure from the top of your head to the tips of your toes.

But where do you go from here? Is it simply a matter of performing every exercise and eating every food I suggested? Or is it better to pick a favored few to which you'll adhere diligently?

The answer is—*neither*. For there is no single, simple course to beauty. Just as occupation, climate, hobby interests and countless other factors determine your individual life-style, so must self-beautifying techniques be custom tailored to your personal needs and goals.

Remember that you are unique—an individual. No one else in the world has your combination of tissues, muscles, skin, hair, mind, and emotions. The grace and charm you achieve are yours alone–inimitable–your trademark.

But remember, too, that you are never the same person you were a year ago, a day ago, even an hour ago. Your body is constantly changing. So are the life you lead, the goals you seek, the needs you encounter.

Clearly, at forty, a woman does not face the same problems she had at twenty. Maturity brings some alterations in physical structure. You must be ready to cope with these changes, not hide from them.

The worst enemy of beauty is fear–the fear of growing old. Too many women still believe that once they reach their middle years, it's all downhill. They see no point in trying to maintain their attractiveness, because they are doomed to creeping infirmity, senility–and ugliness.

Nothing could be further from the truth. Beauty knows no age barriers. It is timeless–and limited only by a woman's negative attitude toward herself. With proper care, your beauty will deepen and mature with the passing years.

Basically, there are four decisive times in life when beauty routines must be reexamined, and, perhaps, restructured:

TEENS TO EARLY TWENTIES
A TIME FOR SEARCHING AND EXPLORATION

Whether you plan to marry early, continue your schooling, or pursue a career, this is your period for developing beauty and health habits. It is your age of self-realization, when you take full responsibility for how you look and feel.

Although you are still young enough to believe that

you will never grow old, now is the time to begin guarding against premature aging:

Moisturize your skin daily—especially around the eyes, knees, and elbows. Deep-cleanse with a facial mask at least once a week.

Explore natural cosmetics and determine which ones best complement your natural loveliness. But don't leap at every newfangled "miracle" cream or lotion that comes along. Read labels—look at prices. You'll be surprised how often the fanciest name brands contain the same ingredients of products that sell at a fraction of their cost.

Discover a sport or vigorous activity which you enjoy. Pursue this pleasurable form of exercise at least three times per week. But—remember at the same time to protect your skin from overexposure.

Learn the values of neatness, cleanliness, good grooming. If necessary, consult a beautician for the hairstyle most complimentary to your facial features. Wash your hair often, and brush vigorously to retain its lustrous, youthful sheen.

MID-TWENTIES TO MID-THIRTIES A PERIOD OF REALIZATION AND ACCOMPLISHMENT

These are critical years, when good beauty investments pay big dividends. But these are also the years when you are tempted to break some of your best long-established beauty habits.

When caring for a family or taking on greater career responsibilities, a woman is often "too busy" to find time for herself. But busy-ness is a poor excuse for letting oneself go to pot.

You must plan your activities more efficiently, making

sure you "budget" in a fixed period, every day, devoted to self-beautification. Remember that time spent on yourself is not a luxury but an investment ... an investment in your future.

It is during this period that your skin starts to settle. The area around the eyes, especially, tends to grow more dry, requiring extra moisturizing.

Take steps to eliminate unnecessary stress and emotional conflicts. When needed, find a quiet spot or warm friend to help you gather your wits and settle your nerves. Get proper rest and relaxation. Take regular vacations and, whenever possible, a day off to rekindle your spirit.

Watch out for those couple of extra pounds sneaking in around arms, waist, and hips. Tummy bulge and thigh fat are also encroaching, while bust muscles are weakening. It is time to start combating these trends with spot exercises.

MID-THIRTIES TO MID-FORTIES AN AGE OF SELF-ASSURANCE

By now you've made it. Whether pursuing a career, a family life, or both, your self-assurance, proper direction, and positive accomplishments have added a whole new character to your looks.

You're in full bloom ... but this is no time to rest on your laurels.

Skin is at a dangerous period, when self-moisturizing slows down. So now you must stimulate and nourish your skin—helping it to shed old cells—with massage, loofahs, and lubricants.

Your hands, which take the greatest punishment of all, need extra care. After each hand chore, apply lubricating creams or lotions—even if you use protective gloves. Exercise the hands and stimulate circulation by rapidly opening and closing the fingers frequently throughout the day. Eliminate brown "liver" spots with a mixture of lemon juice, glycerin and sea salt.

If you've slipped into sedentary living habits, regular exercise is essential—not only for your appearance but for your health as well.

See your dentist regularly to combat tooth decay and, most important, gum disease. Lost teeth, even when replaced by dentures, cause facial muscles to distort and sag.

MID-FIFTIES AND ONWARD
A TIME OF SERENITY AND CELEBRATION

There is an old saying: "At twenty, you have the beauty you inherited, at forty the beauty you developed, at sixty the beauty you deserve."

You've reached the fountainhead of beauty and brilliance. You project the certainty which quietly yet firmly states, "This is me and what I did with my life. I wouldn't change a moment of it. *And there's a whole lot more to come!*"

These could be your very best years, lived with zest and exuberance, if you continue to take pride in your appearance. Dress prettily and stay well-groomed. Don't develop the "housecoat habit."

Grooming is essential. Take more time (now that you can afford it) to make yourself "extra beautiful" each day. Remember, a great many people are your audience, many of them young and impressionable. If they see you letting yourself go, they may follow your lead.

Skin is drying faster now, so your facial foundations should be liquid only—nothing that will cake or crack and make you appear older. You must completely abandon cheap, harsh commercial soaps, which are drying to delicate skin. Cleanse only with special fortified soaps * or cream cleansers.

Winter heating can damage and dry the skin as severely as summer sun. Make certain your home heating system is properly humidified.

Baths and showers can be drying to some skins at this age. If so, cut down to three or four a week—or just enough to maintain normal hygiene. On days when you don't bathe, use a *wet* towel all over the body to remove surface perspiration.

Keep your body limber with regular, mild exercises. Take a leisurely stroll or similar activity every day, if possible.

Poor posture is a disaster at this age. It makes you appear many years older than you really are. Always stand tall, with shoulders back, head up. If correct posture is not maintained, your chin will double, your shoulders will sag, your back will develop a curvature. Hold your back straight, tummy in, buttocks tucked under at all times.

Keep a careful watch over your health. Visit your physician and dentist for regular checkups.

Most of all, do not close the books on yourself. You are still a vibrant, beautiful woman—and everyone should know it. You've earned the right to be a bit of a show-off!

Though your beauty program may undergo many changes during your lifetime, some requirements are constant no matter what your age.

Good health, as I have stressed throughout, is essential to lasting loveliness. Whether you are seventeen or seventy, your outer self must be nourished from within.

* You might consider trying Lelord Kordel's Special Soap, fortified with important beauty elements. It is available in health-food stores.

This means, at all ages, adhering to the elements of proper nutrition: abundant proteins, vitamins, and minerals; cutting down on starches and sugars—even the natural kinds; elimination of the *empty* refined carbohydrates—white flour and white sugar.

Only then will you achieve the most important facet of beauty: inner radiance. It will cause your eyes to shine, your smile to sparkle, your skin to glisten. You will become *totally* lovely.

And therein lies the real secret of beauty—the quality that makes it ageless, timeless. Perhaps that is what the poet John Keats meant when he wrote:

> "A thing of beauty is a joy forever:
> Its loveliness increases; it will never
> Pass into nothingness . . ."

THE END